# CHASING
## THE COSMIC PRINCIPLE

Dowsing from Pyramids to Back Yard America

# ROBERT EGBY

Author of the Award Winning
*The Quest of the Radical Spiritualist*
*INSIGHTS: The Healing Paths of the Radical Spiritualist*
*HOLY DIRT, SACRED EARTH: A Dowser's Journey in New Mexico*

Three Mile Point Publishing
Chaumont, NY

Chasing the Cosmic Principle:
Dowsing from Pyramids to Back Yard America

Copyright © Robert Egby

Published by:
Three Mile Point Publishing
26941 Three Mile Point Road
Chaumont, NY 13622

www.robertegbybooks.com

Basic formatting and cover design by Jera Publishing

First published
Three Mile Point Publishing
September 2016

ISBN: 978-0-984-8664-7-2
Library of Congress Control Number: 2016909778

Printed in the United States of America

## ACKNOWLEDGMENTS

We would like to acknowledge the pioneering work carried out on the geospiral phenomena in the United Kingdom: The late Guy Underwood for *The Pattern of the Past*, the late Dennis Wheatley who wrote *The Essential Dowsing Guide* and his daughter, Maria Wheatley who continues to explore and teach at Avebury and many other ancient sites. Their experiences have helped many dowsers explore the beneficial Earth energies.

The work of Betty Lou Kishler and Ann Chrissley in checking and proofing this manuscript is highly appreciated.

In this work we have attempted to show that leys and geospirals can be found in most parts of the world and this window has been opened to explorers by the facility known as Google Earth. A member of our circle once termed it as a "view from Heaven." Without that availabilty much of this book would not have been written so easily. Google Earth a free service for everyone is much appreciated.

Finally, I would like to express infinite thanks to Bernard for his assistance, perseverance and patience in finding leys and instruction in Blind Dowsing.

# CONTENTS

# INTRODUCTION

There is a lot of fun and learning in tracking down Earth energies and observing how they affect people in places of learning, hospitals and businesses, often without those people being aware. This is not unusual because most people are asleep, a point made almost a century ago by mystical teacher George Gurdjieff. As many dowsers are aware many people live and die on Geopathic Zones completely oblivious of the dangers to their immune systems. Anyway, this is not what this book is about.

The target of this book is to demonstrate that there are abundances of energies called geospirals and leys that spread positive Earth energy in abundance and there is no need to flock to ancient pagan and spiritual centers to find and enjoy them. They may well be in your neighborhood or even your in your back yard. What is more they have been there for centuries, probably millennia.

This study came about after my partner Betty Lou Kishler and I spent many weeks tracking down geospiral energies in New Mexico. We discovered that Native Ancestors led the way in discovery and used them for building their pueblos. As Europeans came and took over by building churches, schools, colleges and communities, the energies attracted many leading edge artists, performers and scholars.

Afterwards, the question arose in our minds, are there leys and geo-spirals in the states around where we live: New York, Pennsylvania and New Jersey? When we stumbled across a geospiral vortex in a remote north country meadow followed by a triple-haired ley line running down an adjoining old railway right of way, we decided to start searching.

At first it was simply going to be a brief study for dowsing workshops, then leys started appearing all over the place — four of them crossing in one town. Then we found a New Jersey town, heavily into academia and there are four leys there. Strange as it may seem schools, colleges, universities, hospitals, health centers, libraries, art centers all seem to cluster on or close to leys which are often accompanied by geospirals.

If it had not been so obvious in New Mexico, it became very obvious in some of the Eastern States. Then two things happened that triggered this book.

One, we started using Google Earth and commenced finding leys and geospirals in the Middle East and Mexico among pyramids and communities there. The other involved the pendulum, one of the strategic instruments of dowsing and the finding of something called the Cosmic Principle.

As we found each energy we researched the background stories and that contributes to this book. Not only that, but dowsers and others interested in the Art and Science of Divining will easily find these places because we noted the geographical coordinates. You might call this work A Dowser's Travel Guide. There are no chapters, but a lot of stories and places to find energy. There are no maps simply because they are prohibitvely expensive. So if you need one obtain an atlas or work with Google Earth.

My view of dowsing is that it is not enough to wave a rod or swing a pendulum and say we found a ley or a geospiral, because there is always a history, a story of it being there. We have explored so little and there is so much to be done. So pick up the tools and explore. You will not regret the adventure.

Robert and Betty Lou
Chaumont New York
June 2016

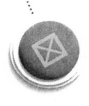

# BOOK ONE

## DISCOVERING THE ENERGIES

No idling about, let us begin. On a large note pad or a regular letter sized blank sheet of paper, write the numerals one to ten, leaving a one to two inch space between each. Then with one hand hold a pendulum above the paper and gently get the weight swinging in a clockwise rotation.

Now with the other hand place your forefinger on number one and watch the swinging pendulum. Wait for a few seconds, then move to number two, keeping the pendulum swinging. Eventually you will get to number nine.

Now watch as the pendulum hesitates, then suddenly changes direction and swings counter-clockwise. Wait for a few seconds while it builds up speed and you may find you are unable to hold the pendulum. Quickly stop it and go to number 10 and the pendulum will suddenly revert to swinging clockwise.

You have just learned how to tune in to something we call the Cosmic Principle. Even if you write the numbers as text, nine will still perform.

Number nine incidentally, even without a pendulum is known to demonstrate strange numerical and mathematical powers. For instance if you multiply any number by nine, it will always return to a nine. Nine times nine equals 81. Eight plus one is nine.

Another: Take our standard numerical system and add each one: $1 + 2 + 3 + 4 + 5 + 6 + 7 + 8 + 9$. The total is 45. Now add four and five and the answer is nine.

Nine is a cosmic number and a principle.

The pendulum reacting counterclockwise is not magic, it is not witchcraft. It is not religious so relax because there is no mob waiting to burn you at the stake. This is an energy process inherent in certain objects and certain designs with which we live every day and strangely most people have no idea about it and if they do hear it mentioned, fail to give it any credence. Most people walking the planet know even less about the powers manifesting on Earth which they call home and which is also a part of the Cosmos. We are not talking science. The word is Consciousness.

Our investigation had simple beginnings. During one of our early morning walks when the dew was still on the grass that flanks an old railroad right-of-way in Northern New York, Betty Lou felt drawn to a remote meadow. A rolling grass filled saucer-shaped depression the size of two football fields was enclosed by tall sentinel oaks and thick undergrowth.

"There's a distinct presence here," she said. "I feel it every time we walk by."

The energy felt similar to that we had experience in New Mexico. Geospirals! Using one rod I asked the question and received an immediate response.

"Is there more than one?"

Immediate reply in the affirmative.

"Show me the alpha."

The search rod swung into the center of the meadow and we started walking. After about forty yards the rod suddenly swung about and pointed in the opposite direction. We had struck center.

It turned out to be the maximum size of geospirals — 49 rings.

There were eleven geospirals in the nest, nine of them in the meadow and two on the railway right-of-way. For the next little while we did what one does best when there is a big collection of geospirals — hang out. It felt good to be there. One's whole body gets to relax. Any appointments or immediate plans are forgotten as one allows the energy to pervade every muscle, every bone, every organ, every gland, every cell in the body. We made a decision to come back with blankets and soak up this beautiful energy. When we did, we discovered something else — a ley line running along the right-of-way where the railway track used to be. This discovery would later lead us to an international energy connection.

Thinking back about the meadow it was much like the energy we found in New Mexico. The Taos Indian pueblo, in the Cathedral Basilica of St. Francis of Assisi at Sante Fe and Los Alamos, the home town of the National Research Laboratory where during World War II they created the first atomic bomb. Geospirals are not judgmental, they simply work to provide an energy that is beneficial to the human body and mind for healing, relaxation and inspiration.

The dowsing rods indicated that the meadow had been a summer camp for Native Ancestors, so it was then I realized that a book was needed to describe these energies simply because Yin energies are beneficial to the human body and its environment. What is more, they are totally FREE and inexhaustible.

Leys have long reigned in my life as a dowser but the phenomenon known as geospirals only surfaced in conducting research for my book *Holy Dirt, Sacred Earth: A Dowser's Journey in New Mexico*. We spent a whole month in 2011 based in Taos and other shorter visits were spread over several years prior to that. Northern New Mexico is a researcher's paradise for the study of how Earth energies impacted and attracted the lives of so many extraordinary and ordinary people.

After reading various books on geospiral research in the United Kingdom that involved Stonehenge, Avebury, Westminster Abbey, Glastonbury and the like, one is inclined to believe that geospiral energy is limited to such ancient and holy venues. After our New Mexico studies it dawned on us that geospirals and leys are much in evidence all over the world.

More important, a whole lot of people were totally aware of them and used them beneficially for themselves and communities. These include

William Penn, Pierre Charles L'Enfant, George Washington, Dr. Edward Trudeau, Rev. Russell Conwell, Compte Pierre Francois Real, George C. Boldt and more. They designed and built schools, libraries, churches, cathedrals, hospitals, research centers and universities and even a whole city on Earth energies such as leys and geospirals. Critics might claim they are coincidences but those who chase the Cosmic Principle smile and move on.

We must not forget the Native Ancestors, the Indian Tribes who were fully aware of leys and geospirals. They walked and lived within the energies and respected them as sacred.

Sacred? As you will see the word is Cosmic. Spirals not only exist on Earth but are found in profusion in many parts of the Great Cosmos.

A point of caution. There are some techniques offered in this book that should only be used by trained dowsers and people who feel totally comfortable with themselves and their powers of imagery. These too create intriguing questions as will be seen. Our mission in creating this report is to discover answers. That is why it is entitled *Chasing the Cosmic Principle: Dowsing from Pyramids to Back Yard America.*

# DOWSING THE EARTH ENERGY

America! Some say it's all a dream, an Eldorado, wealth for the taking. Others see it as a nightmare, a dark land of fears, gunslingers and threats to one's life.

America is a manufactured nation, wrestling between twenty million living at or below the poverty line and the modern-day caesars, corporate moguls scheming and battling to achieve greater profits where a couple of million bucks is pocket money.

Then there are the ordinary folks who mechanically perform their daily lives perhaps broken by an occasional dream of a vacation on a tropical beach, or simply sitting in front of a mega-screen watching endless sports while feeding an interminable thirst for beer and chips.

As Georges Gurdjieff suggested well over a century ago: "People are asleep." They either dwell on things past or worry about security in the mists of an uncertain future.

When the gurus chant: Live Now, the peace that comes with living in the present is too difficult to understand let alone practice. Few wish to consider there is another side to the great land.

It can be called Mysterious America, a land that has been largely forgotten in the hectic days of 21ˢᵗ century living. It is a land full of strange energies that attract, guide, heal and enlighten or challenge one's spirituality and beliefs. Many energies one can see and feel are like sunshine, the cold winds of winter, heat from the fire, the touch of a loved one. But there are many energies flowing rapidly through a home to which the occupants may be completely oblivious. Examples: radio and broadcast signals, wireless phone calls, microwaves, and energies projected by electrical wires running through the walls. They are all there and you cannot in your normal mode of being see or feel them or even pay much attention..

For the unaware, there are energies that can kill and there are energies that can heal, inspire and rejuvenate.

It is safe to say most people are totally unaware of the abundant natural energies that exist around and within. Our American ancestors, the Indians, were fully aware and fully conscious of these energies. They respected, learned and worked with them. But so did the so called ancient civilizations all over the planet.

# THE ANCIENT ART OF DOWSING

Most dowsing can be accomplished by using any of the following: two L-shaped copper rods, a forked willow branch, a pendulum or any small weight attached to a piece of string. One ancient Egyptian method that surfaces frequently in drawings and carvings depicts a wand or stick to which ribbons or long leaves are attached. My late friend and colleague, veteran Canadian dowser Tom Passey frequently used the remains of a fine fly-fishing rod, minus the reel and about a meter in length.

Dowsing started early among the shrouds of mists of surrounding human origins. Someone, somewhere on the great plains of life discovered that if one cut a stick and tied some fine vine leaves to the end, the leaves would quiver when they were near ground water and again if the gathering clouds would bring rain. Life progressed and the rod became adorned with loose ribbons that trembled ecstatically when water or certain rocks or animals were present. These can be viewed in Egyptian hieroglyphics, wall paintings in caves, manuscripts and ancient sites. Others tied a small weight to a piece of string and found similar results and so the pendulum swung into life.

Thus the noble art of dowsing and divining was born. It became the secret and prized art of the magi, the priests, the wizards, the medicine men and women and indeed the heads of tribes because it possessed a "power." Followers unable to comprehend called them wands because the wooden rods seemed to work magic.

In the Tassili n'Ajjer caves in south-east Algeria near the borders of Libya, Niger and Mali there are thousands of incredible wall paintings of wildlife, but there is also a picture of a dowser, holding a forked branch in his hands while being watched by tribal people. Carbon dating has set the paintings at over 8,000 years old.

Ancient Egyptian temples show pictographs of pharaohs with sticks resembling dowsing rods that date two millennia BCE. A Cairo museum contains pendulums well over 1,000 years old.

Whenever the ancients required something they simply resorted to their rods or their pendulums. They never lacked for water, never lost their way, and the divining rod always answered. Their rods and pendulums became their personal oracles and they never went far without them. Such words in Psalm 23 confirm this: *Thy rod and thy staff shall comfort me.*

Back in biblical history Moses used a rod, otherwise known as a staff to perform dowsing which is related in Numbers 20: "and Moses and Aaron gathered the assembly before the rock. And he said to them, 'Listen now, you rebels; shall we bring forth water for you out of this rock?' Then Moses lifted up his hand and struck the rock twice with his rod; and water came forth abundantly, and the congregation and their beasts drank."

In the old days dowsing was called water-witching and in medieval times regardless of what Moses and other great teachers and biblical figures did, dowsing was frequently branded "ungodly" and practitioners were liable to be tortured and even burned at the stake.

The man who triggered this and made it very unhealthy was Emperor Theodosius who used the newly formed Universal Catholic Church and the flag of Christianity to close down and crush pagan temples, oracles, healing centers and such gathering places from one end of the Roman Empire to the other.

Spirit communicators, diviners, healers and orators were captured and exiled, imprisoned or executed. It was a condemnation that lasted almost a thousand years and even in the last century mediums and healers were still being imprisoned because of so-called Christian principles that had nothing to do with Jesus, but due to Roman emperors.

The British Witchcraft Act of 1735 remained in force well into the 20th century until its eventual repeal with the enactment of the Fraudulent Mediums Act of 1951. Incidentally it was only repealed as recently as May 26th 2008 simply by pressures brought by the European Union laws which targeted "unfair sales and marketing practices." In South Africa the Witchcraft Suppression law based on the original British Act of 1735 is still in force although it is currently (2015) under review.

It is always best to remember that if all the prophets and spiritual leaders mentioned in the Holy Bible, including Moses, Jesus and the Apostles were alive just a few years ago, they would be lucky to be just serving prison sentences. Such were the dictatorial powers of Emperor Theodosius and the controls of newly formed Universal Catholic Church.

Today, divining through dowsing, water witching, intuiting and higher consciousness is alive and well and practiced through many countries of the world helping people improve their daily lives and also to open minds to higher awareness and consciousness. One still cannot understand why such arts and skills are not taught in our schools.

Simply put dowsing is the skill of finding targets, visible and invisible, using the power of the Higher Consciousness. We are going to use this skill to discover Earth energies, their values and their impact on people and more.

# THE INSTRUMENTS OF POWER

The pilgrim needs four things to understand and work with the subjects explored on this journey.

- A human body with an open minded Higher Consciousness and an acute desire to learn;
- A pair of L-rods.
- A Pendulum.
- Maps, maps and more maps.
- With these attributes the pilgrim can explore everything from a flock of pyramids in the Nubian Desert, an energy line running through Congress in Washington D.C., a geospiral behind a local church or a deadly geopathic zone running through a loved one's bedroom.

I forgot to mention: In this day and age it is good strategy to have a good sized laptop equipped with a program called *Google Earth*.

Google Earth? It is a great system in the Digital Age. Worry not, it is easy to use and as the pilgrim will see, it is possible to dowse any energy on any plot of land anywhere on Earth. This is discussed in detail under Digital Dowsing. For now we are talking pendulums.

# SELECTING THE "RIGHT" PENDULUM

It happens. When you are about to seek a pendulum you will find yourself asking a veteran how do I find the right pendulum? The reply will often be like this: "Use a pendulum to find a pendulum."

Well, that was like the other twisted statement, what came first the chicken or the egg? However it does have an element of truth. Once you have the knack or the talent of using a pendulum it will be easy to discover another pendulum suited to your psyche.

A pendulum is defined as an object — a bob — suspended by a fine chain or string so that it swings freely back and forth under the influence of gravity. In practical terms you can use just about anything: a metal nut, key, nail or bolt attached to a fine chain or tied on the end of a piece of string will create a basic pendulum. A ring, a pendant or brooch on a fine chain will do nicely. Most serious dowsers use crystals, polished stones and small brass knobs that come in various shapes and sizes. Traditionally in working with maps and charts it is convenient to have a pendulum with a sharp point.

There was a dowser in our Canadian group who used a .22 caliber bullet hanging on a chain and when accosted by strangers replied: "What better use to put ammunition than in a pendulum for dowsing."

Traditional map and chart dowsers find it convenient to use a pendulum with a sharp point which is excellent if you have papers and documents. My way is different because I mainly use digital laptop maps for which I use a sharp but harmless pointer on the screen and hold a pendulum in my right hand. My pendulum is a well worn brass knob on a chain that came from an old electric lamp. You see, any small object on a string or chain can act as a pendulum. It serves me well. A discussion on digital map reading is forthcoming.

# UNLIMITED HORIZONS OF DOWSING

By the way, dowsing has unlimited possibilities. For instance, a pendulum can be used to find directions, ask the time, check the energy of a house or an apartment you might be going to rent or purchase, discover how the weather will be on a certain date in the future, the wisdom of starting a business or economic project, enrolling in an education course and much more.

In health and welfare matters, dowsing will reveal the amount of calories on a plate of food, and determine the fat content. You can even check the nutritional content of food and if you have a list of vitamins and minerals, you can check your own or a friend's body for vitamin and mineral balance. Another favorite of dowsers is checking the sex of an unborn child.

With a pendulum you can, always with permission, scan a friend's body and determine a past history of surgical operations, bone breakages, organ and gland weaknesses, plus energy blockages that need to be resolved. Arthritis, a stress related disease, has a habit of originating in areas where old bone breakages occurred many years ago. Pendulums are great for tracking body and auric energies. Many naturopaths and other health professionals use pendulums for tracking the roots of physical ailments.

In metaphysics there are a number of power centers in the human body. These are known as chakras and a pendulum will tell you if they are correctly aligned or out of balance and by what percentage.

One other point, some geological exploration companies employ professional dowsers with maps to assist in finding locations for oil, gas, minerals, water, precious metals, archeological remains and even undersea treasures. This has occurred several times off the coast of Egypt, particularly Alexandria where various ruins lie at the bottom of the Mediterranean. For the most part dowsers perform their work without leaving the office. This facility is termed map dowsing and we sometimes use this technique for finding geospirals and ley lines in remote locations where prolonged travel is difficult or near impossible.

## HOW DOES IT WORK EXACTLY?

Ah, there's the rub. Dowsing fraternity members will offer a variety of answers. Some claim the pendulum swing is triggered by a very fine neuromuscular reaction triggered by the Higher Self. Others claim it is a psychic ability but this is spurned by true blooded dowsers. Some say the whole thing works on universal or earth energy. One point is definite: There must always be a human element. Pendulums and dowsing rods do not work by themselves, yet. When a robot equipped with AI — artificial intelligence — comes along and does the work, a whole lot of dowsers will hang up their pendulums and rods.

For my part, I believe dowsing is the manifestation of higher consciousness working in conjunction with the sub-conscious mind which answers through neuromuscular reaction. It is the metaphysical part of our being, the intuitive sense, the sixth sense that is in tune with Universal Consciousness.

## HOLDING THE PENDULUM

The most practical way of holding the pendulum's chain is with the forefinger and thumb of your strong hand — that's your writing hand. Some dowsers advise using the weak or non-writing hand. The bottom line is whatever works for you — do it!.

Let the pendulum hang loosely. Some people fancy longer chains, about twelve inches, others like it to be two or three inches. Remember, a shorter chain or string creates a faster response. Start with a twelve inch chain and discover your own preferred and ideal working length. My personal preference is three inches and when working in a strong breeze, one inch. Yes, passing breezes can block a long chain or string.

## CARING FOR A PENDULUM

Once you are equipped with the right pendulum, get a pouch or soft cloth container and keep it as you would a valuable gift. Do not allow anyone else to use it, no matter if they are the most angelic and trustworthy person in the world. If you think your pendulum might have been exposed to negative energy, place it on a piece of cloth and expose it to sunshine for several days. If you are in a hurry, you can wash it in salty sea water or apple cider vinegar. Both are great for cleansing pendulums from unwanted energies. Make sure your pendulum is safe for cleaning. If in doubt, use the sunshine mode.

A pendulum should always be kept and carried in a protected place.

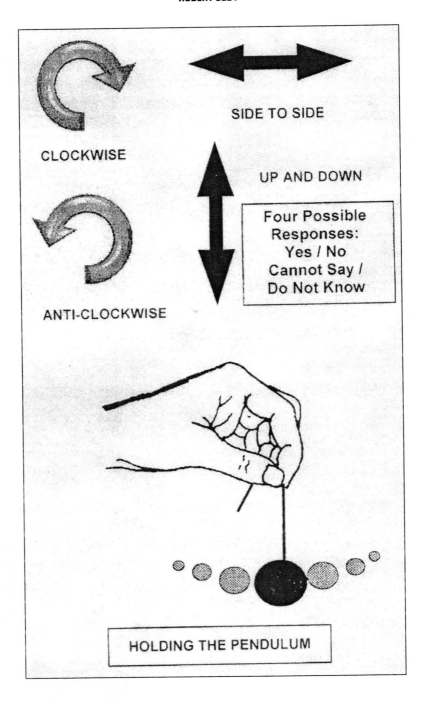

CLOCKWISE

SIDE TO SIDE

UP AND DOWN

ANTI-CLOCKWISE

Four Possible
Responses:
Yes / No
Cannot Say /
Do Not Know

HOLDING THE PENDULUM

# THREE OR FOUR RESPONSES?

It all depends on whom you ask whether there are three or four responses obtainable from a swinging pendulum. I teach four responses, my old friend and colleague, Canadian Tom Passey used to teach three. Again, it is whatever works for you.

My four responses are: YES, NO, CAN'T SAY, and DON'T KNOW. The last two responses are based on (1) your higher consciousness refusing to tell you, and (2) the higher consciousness simply does not know the answer probably because the question is ambiguous. Ambiguity in forming a question is the bane of people learning to dowse. Be blunt and direct for what you are seeking. It pays.

The first two responses from a pendulum are fairly straight forward. My YES is a circular clockwise movement of the pendulum, and the NO is an counter-clockwise circle. Yours may be different.

My CANNOT SAY is a straight back and forth, and my DO NOT KNOW is like a shaking of the head, side to side movement. Please check the attached diagram.

# EXERCISE — LEARNING TO SWING

Never hurry dowsing or anything else in metaphysics including meditation. Dowsing is very much like meditation so stay cool and relaxed. Take time out to close your eyes and slowly take several deep breaths. Alternatively close your eyes and imagine you can look up inside your forehead for five to ten seconds. Either of these techniques will place you in a comfortable altered state of consciousness — in other words, relaxed.

Your arm should be free. Resist the desire to rest on a table or against your body. In fact, many dowsers suggest the arm should be a little tired, much like an arm used in automatic writing. First, give the pendulum a gentle motivating swing then generally keep your hand still after that.

- First, address the pendulum: "When I ask a question and the answer is YES show me the response that means YES." Now, when you have an affirmative response, bring the pendulum back to a slight swinging mode.
- This time ask your pendulum to: "When I ask a question and the answer is NO show me the response that means NO." Now, when you have a negative response, bring the pendulum back to a slight swinging mode.
- Next, do as above but address your pendulum as follows: "When I ask a question and the answer is CANNOT SAY show me the response that means "CANNOT SAY."
- Finally, to your pendulum say: "When I ask a question and the answer is DO NOT KNOW, show me the "DO NOT KNOW" response.

Keep practicing until you get all four responses. They may be weak at first with the pendulum hardly moving but with practice the responses become stronger. When you feel comfortable and everything is working do this simple test.

## TESTING YOUR PENDULUM

Prepare your pendulum by allowing it to swing gently in neutral. Start a session with *"May I ask a question at this time?"* It is blunt and direct. Some dowsers ask their pendulums: *"May I? Can I ? Should I? ask a question?"* It is your choice. Wait for a response and if the pendulum swings affirmatively, perform the following test.

*"Is my name......?"* Pick the name of someone else. The response should be a negative.

Now use your correct name. The response should be in the affirmative.

Once you have established this you are ready to venture forth and get some dowsing practice. However, do refrain from getting excited, stressed or hurried. Pendulums and your higher consciousness are averse to fluctuating energies. But as Tom Passey advised in countless workshops: *"Practice! Practice! Practice!"* Many people neglect to perform this point.

Experience is vital to good and effective dowsing and experience comes through practice. If you desire to become an accomplished pianist, you must practice. Likewise if you wish to be a good skier, tennis player, mathematician, floral arranger, photographer, speaker, actor, psychic or healer, you must practice; so it is with dowsing. Practice with real energies at every opportunity you get. Encourage them. Beg for them. Enjoy and appreciate your trials and errors because they are all valuable learning experiences.

# WORKING WITH THE L-RODS

If you are searching for geospirals and earth energies of any sort it is advisable to be proficient in the use of L-rods. An excellent point about L-rods is that they normally come in pairs but you can always use one doubling up as a pendulum or as a search tool.

The L-rod looks like an L with the lower base forming the handle and the upright section of the L making the pointer. In the search position the two pointing arms are parallel, and when they reach the target they either become crossed or fly apart. Rods range in length from about three inches to 18 inches. The longer ones are more difficult to manipulate on windy days.

The American Society of Dowsers, the British Society of Dowsers, the Canadian Society of Dowsers along with independent suppliers carry a variety of L-rods ranging from simple pieces of wire to sophisticated ones with wooden or brass handles. If you are talented and work inclined, they are easy to make with strong wire such as bronzed welding rods, a small vice, a pair of wire cutters and pliers.

Copper coat-hangers make good dowsing rods as well. Cut two usable pieces, perhaps 18 or 20 inches in length. Bend a length of five inches for your handle, so that the wire forms an L. Next acquire two empty pen casings and slip them over the handles, then with pliers bend the bottom of the handles so the casings do not fall off. Because the arms may be sharp, slip small protective caps on the ends. The last thing you need is a sharp stabbing by your own dowsing rods.

# HOLDING THE L-RODS

There are two photos in this section showing the search position for the L-rods. The search position for using L-rods is to stand holding the handles in front of your chest with the arms pointing forward towards the horizon. You can imagine you're holding two six-guns like an old time gunfighter, but after lots of years practice I find gently holding the handles with your thumbs and fingers is the best. To be in a search position the rods should point to a place just below the horizon.

# CRITICAL POINTS: FOCUS AND IMAGERY

In anything you want in life, it is best achieved by being focused and so it is in dowsing. Focus on your target. Regardless of whether you are using pendulums or rods, the dowser must be able to concentrate and focus on the object which is the subject of his or her search.

In your mind visualize the objective. For instance if you are looking for a geospiral, fix that image in your mind before you go into the search position. See it clearly in your mind and if any other thoughts slip in, gently push them out. Your subconscious mind will soon catch onto this important search habit.

If you cannot focus well, relax and perform this excellent training exercise. Find a clock with a second hand. Sit in front and observe the movement of the second hand for 60 seconds. If any thoughts pop into your mind, gently move them away and refocus. Do this several times over several days and you will find your powers of concentration improve dramatically.

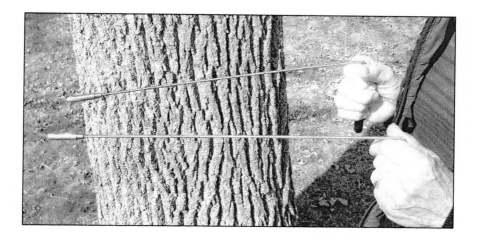

Dowsing rods in the Search Position

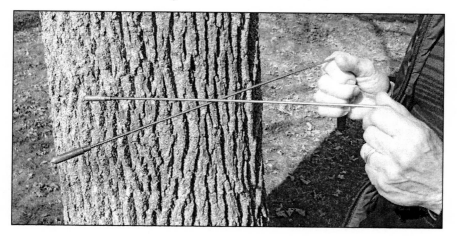

Dowsing rods crossed at the Target.

# THE SEARCH POSITION

Hold the handles of both L-rods as described above. Walk slowly with both rod pointers parallel and aiming gently down, a few degrees below the horizon. Focus on the object of the search. For a test: search for the edges of a shadow or the underground pipes of a lawn watering system. Or have a person stand still and ask for the edge of that person's aura. The rods should cross or swing wide apart the moment you reach the target.

Resist a display of emotional joy, amazement or the desire to throw a party. Rods and pendulums are averse to such emotional storms. Stay cool and perform another test.

# ENERGY LINES TO KNOW

### GEOPATHIC LINES

This is a phenomenon you need to know as a dowser but it really does not come up in this study. Planet Earth radiates a constant beneficial and healthy force, however when this energy passes through divisions in rock or subterranean water veins with a clay base it makes a 180 degree phase change from positive to negative.

If humans and animals spend prolonged periods on a geopathic zone, such as sleeping or working at a desk, the negative force reduces the human immune system. Its impact or influence affects people not immediately but over weeks and sometimes several months. Victims begin to suffer physically and/or mentally and often receive medical treatments that fail to help. Prolonged exposure can mean death. An excellent description of some 11,000 cases conducted by European dowser Käthe Bachler's are given in her classic book *Earth Radiation*.

A surefire way of recognizing symptoms of a geopathic zone occurs in nearby trees. A tree standing on a geopathic zone may become distorted. Bark is twisted, gnarled and may even have ugly knots protruding in different places. The trees appear in pain — and they are. On the other hand trees standing on positive energy such as geospirals and leys are normally thick and abundant and that subject is coming up shortly.

## LEY LINES OR "OLD TRACKS"

Planet Earth is laced with a strange and mysterious phenomena known as ley lines. There is no rhyme nor reason for them but they are extraordinarily useful to animals and humankind.

Normally a ley comes as a single line or hair and may cover a few miles. Occasionally they manifest in three lines or hairs, in which case we refer to them as triple-haired leys. There is really no set length for leys. One might go hundreds of miles while another might run a mere mile. The only constant is they exist in straight lines, even when crossing water such as lakes, rivers and oceans. According to lunar movements they appear to intensify at full moon and again at new moon but these movements are minimal. In addition they have been found to move a few feet but they do return. A dowser once suggested that ley lines are being projected on the planet from outer space. No one appears to have come up with any further information.

The Ancient Native Ancestors were fully aware and utilized leys in various ways mainly for travel in migration or simply to journey from one community or hunting ground to another.

Dowsers can become quite sensitive to leys from frequent searching, measuring and aligning. For instance, Betty Lou and I were in a birdseed shop and I happened to be holding a dangling pendulum at my side. Suddenly it began rapidly swirling around and I realized we were standing on a ley. The strange thing is I was not looking or thinking about leys. Anyway the discovery turned out to be a major ley running across New Jersey into Pennsylvania. A weird discovery brought about by an alert Higher Consciousness.

While ley lines existed and certain people knew of them and for security reasons maintained a tight cloak of secrecy, it was not until 1921 when an English flour mill owner and avid photographer took notice. Alfred Watkins was riding his horse in Hertfordshire, a county north of London, when he noticed that many of the foot paths and lanes seemed to connect one hilltop to another in a straight line. He subsequently coined the term "ley" because the lines passed through places whose names contained the syllables "ley, lay, lea, lee, or leigh."

In an intensive study of maps he noticed that key points were in alignment. For instance churches built on old pagan or Celtic spiritual sites appeared mysteriously in a line.

"The whole thing came to me in a flash," he later told his son. Watkins subsequently found ley lines that connected standing stones, ancient earthworks, stone monuments and circles, cairns, megaliths, barrows and sites of ancient towns and villages. In his book, *Early British Trackways* published in 1922, he describes his various findings. The book triggered a new movement among archaeologists, hikers and of course dowsers.

Suddenly historical events were shown in a new light. Leys were used by ancient Britons to move from one community to another. They sensed the energy or they followed the stone markers.

Following Watkins's revelations British dowsers quickly found major leys in Glastonbury, Stonehenge, Avebury, St. Michael's Mount, and in major cities. For instance at the Gothic Westminster Abbey in London a leyline runs directly east-west through the ancient structure and it is flanked by nests of geospirals all radiating Yin energy.

Many dowsers are aware of the major line known as the St. Michael's Ley that rises out of the Atlantic and passes through St. Michael's Mount in Cornwall. It crosses many historic places such as Bodmin, Glastonbury, Devizes, Luton and on to Bury St. Edmonds and Hopton-on-Sea in Norfolk before disappearing into the North Sea. It was originally labeled the Great Dragon Line, mainly because St. Michael the patron saint of fishermen slew a dragon terrorizing fishermen.

Back in the early 1980s I hiked sections of this ley and discovered that even without dowsing rods you can sense the earth energy manifesting in your body. Therefore I could well imagine our ancient ancestors walking along these lines as they traveled from one place to another.

St. Michael's Ley possesses many churches named after the saint and they dot the hills along the ley where once stood pagan circles, temples and places of worship. Christians loved to build their worshiping centers on old pagan sacred sites.

# LEYS A PREHISTORIC GPS SYSTEM

When one starts to investigate this form of energy it often appears like a prehistoric Global Positioning System aka GPS. An alert hiker or dowser may well observe cattle in the meadows walking along certain tracks towards their feed or barn. For the most part they all follow invisible lines and if you dowse them you are more than likely to find ley lines — the old tracks. This actually occurs in many other countries including the United States and Canada.

Since Watkins' time considerable work has been conducted by dowsers in mapping leylines that criss-cross England, Wales and Scotland. In more recent times, the term ley line has come to be associated with spiritual and mystical theories about land forms, including Chinese feng shui, a point made by John Michell in his book *The New View over Atlantis.*

In Egypt the Great Pyramid at Giza is a focal point for many leys and they intensify its latent and Cosmic energy. Whoever created the great monument knew exactly what he or she was doing from global and energy points of view. The ancient pyramid builders did not create a vortex in Egypt, it was already there and they simply recognized one as a cosmic crossroads, enjoyed the energy and used it to their own ends.

But the power of the ley is not restricted to Europe, the Middle East and South America, there is a multiplicity of leys in the United States and Canada and pioneers from the Native Ancestors to the early European settlers based their communities on them. These include Philadelphia, Princeton, New York and Washington DC. If someone claims none of them were dowsed it is clearly an untruth based on ignorance as the streets and buildings stand directly on ley lines. Coincidence is not an option. How they came about is discussed in chapters ahead.

Leys and geospirals are often found together, but the link appears coincidental, because there is no strict rule that they must exist together, in fact geospirals can and are found individually in gardens, parks, fields and places many miles from any ley activity.

There is one observation at this point: both leys and geospirals transmit Yin energies which complement each other, intensifying the joint Area of Influence.

Finding leys is extremely easy. If you think or feel there is one near to your home or office, stand with one L-rod and adopt a search mode. Presumably you will have primed your instrument with "May I ask a question?" you say "Show me the nearest ley," or "Point to the nearest ley." When the rod stops follow the direction until it suddenly swings about. You have just struck your target.

# THE GEOSPIRAL PHENOMENA

Spirals are everywhere. NASA tells us that spirals make up approximately 60 percent of the galaxies in our local universe. Ancient cultures around the world left petroglyphs or rock engravings plus cave paintings that frequently display spirals. This raises the question did they intuitively guess the enormous numbers of spiral galaxies in the Cosmic heavens or were they told about them by ancient astronauts such as those referred to in the Cuneiform tablets from Sumeria.?

Or did they dowse their sacred places and discover energy spirals emanating from underground waters and figure out these must also be found out there in the Cosmos? It just seems very strange that so many spiritual and sacred monuments around the world are or were built on blind springs or water domes that manifest spiraling energy fields that we call geospirals.

Blind springs are fed by water streams produced deep within the Earth and are forced by high pressure through geological faults towards the surface. Sometimes the water emerges as springs and occasionally meets impenetrable horizontal rock strata where it becomes blocked or domed until it finds outlets. In the process it produces invisible but powerful energy forces known as geospirals.

British archaeologist and Master Dowser the late Guy Underwood is recognized as the modern day discoverer or re-discoverer of the phenomena. He spent many years in the 1930s and 1940s researching geospirals and explains the findings in intricate detail in his classic book *The Pattern of the Past*. Excellent additional work has been done by British dowsers the late Dennis Wheatley of Swindon and his daughter Maria Wheatley of Avebury.

Mr. Wheatley described the geospiral as one of the geodetic system's "most exotic geometric patterns."

Geospirals manifest energy circles in many sizes. Some can be as small as a few paces — five to ten feet, while some, according to Mr. Underwood range over hundreds of feet. The largest spirals we have discovered ranged over some 140 feet.

A geospiral is measured by its coils or rings and strangely they are counted in sevens — the smallest being a seven. The others are 14, 21, 28, 35, 42 and 49 rings.

If a dowser goes to Stonehenge in England for example, the Altar Stone will show a seven ring geospiral while the Heel Stone will display a 49 ring spiral.

Geospirals rarely come singly, in fact the majority come in nests of five and more. The most we have experienced is a nest of 19 on an old French church site at Rosiere, NY.

One peculiarity: Geospirals frequently overlap one another and when this occurs the Area of Influence expands as well, making the area in the vicinity very attractive for relaxation, healing, meditation, creative thought and spiritual activities including spirit communication.

The energy from a geospiral is not only lateral, it is vertical as well and appears to represent a dome or a set of domes.

## DOWSING THE GEOSPIRAL:

Sure-fire places for finding geospirals are historically sacred places such as monasteries, cathedrals, ancient burial grounds, pueblos, pyramids and more. The problem is caretakers, supervisors, gatekeepers frequently get upset not because they are opposed to dowsing but they fear negative reaction from sightseers. That is why some dowsers at high visibility places carry miniature dowsing rods, three inches long, just in case.

But let us make it loud and clear there are many other places, sometimes obscure and tucked away where geospirals operate in relative secrecy. There may be some in your local park, a meadow or even in your own yard. If you know where Native Indians built their villages or held summer camps, test them out. They always built on geospirals and considered them sacred.

## STARTING THE SEARCH:

Set a rod in the search position and ask if there are any geospirals within a short distance — 100 or two hundred yards of where you are standing. If the reply is in the affirmative, ask for the alpha, the leader of the nest. The rod will probably change direction, in which case follow it until it suddenly swings about and points the way you have come. You have found the geospiral center.

The next step is to measure the rings. Start at the center and holding both L-rods in the parallel search position walk away from the center. The rods will cross every time you walk over a ring and then immediately swing back into the search position. Count the number of times this happens - 7, 14, 21, 28, 35, 42 and 49 — and you have the power of the geospiral.

Do not rest upon your laurels. Check for additional geospirals. Ask the search rod if there are other geospirals in the immediate area. If it points to a new location, call it "Geospiral 2". When you have reached that, ask for Geospiral 3 and so on. You may well find there are six or even nine geospirals in the area, in which case you have a minor vortex.

In order to keep your sanity on where each one exists and how many there are, use simple yellow or orange markers. These are little landscaping flags on sticks that can be acquired at almost any hardware store. Place one in the center of each spiral. This technique will present a layout of the geospiral nest. Take a photograph or make a map and note the number of rings of each one.

At this point you may wish to use a pendulum and measure the depth and capacity of the blind spring underneath your feet.

## MEASURING THE AREA OF INFLUENCE:

Now when you discover a large collection stand at the alpha geospiral and say: "I wish to measure the area of influence of these geospirals. Please cross the rods when I reach the edge of the area. Commence walking. You may be amazed to find it may be a quarter or even half a mile or more. The Blue Lake geospiral vortex at Taos, New Mexico radiates for several miles but does change with the weather and moon.

Another, less physically draining method of finding the edge of an Area of Influence is to use a pendulum and suggest different distances until you get a positive answer.

## BEWARE! THEY ARE ALIVE!

Geospirals have irregularities: You may mark the center of one on one day and bring friends to see it the next day and find it has moved several feet. So you re-stake it and return another day only to discover it is back at the original position. Geospirals are living phenomena.

## TREES ON GEOSPIRALS:

Something we have discovered is that when a tree grows over a geospiral the tree sprouts several strong and healthy trunks all blossoming from one point. In Northern New York there are frequent examples. One flanks the old Watertown-Cape Vincent railway track and has seven trunks all big and strong and not malformed like they would be if growing on a geopathic zone. The positive energy emanating from geospirals encourages plant and tree growth.

## THE MOVING CAR SEARCH METHOD:

One method of finding geospirals is for the dowser to sit as a passenger in a moderately moving car (20-30 mph) with one L-rod. Ask to the rod to indicate any geospirals within a quarter of a mile. As you travel along you will find the rod starting to pick up geospiral activity in the distance and then swing round as you pass. Make a note of any cross roads and return to the area on foot and using one L-rod walk in the direction indicated.

That is how we found the one in the town of Brownville just outside Watertown, NY. The Universalist Church started in 1854 and after becoming defunct, the building in 1900 became the Catholic Church of the Immaculate Conception. We stopped the car and found a geospiral just in front of the church altar.

The moving car method helps the enquiring dowser find geospirals over a much larger area. Just do not drive and dowse. A rod might get bent out of shape.

## LIVING WITH A GEOSPIRAL:

People living on or near a geospiral may encounter problems. While we have some idea of the benefits of temporary exposure to a geospiral, we are still surveying families living within the Area of Influence of a geospiral or have one in their backyard.

In Marlton NJ there is a family with a small geospiral in their front yard. It came to light while searching for a geopathic zone that the family believed was negatively affecting the home. There was indeed a geopathic zone cutting across one part of the house close to where a baby slept so we cleared that then asked: "Are there any geospirals at this location?" The rod swung round to the front yard.

Here's a rule which I think dowsers should follow: When searching for geopathic/negative zones always check to see if there are any geospirals affecting the property. While geospial energy is good, too much can disrupt lives.

The mother at the Marlton house told us: "We have all the children's toys located at the back of the house but they keep bringing them to the front yard and playing with them there," she said. "Always!"

The spot? Exactly on the center of the geospiral.

It was only a seven ring phenomenon but its area of influence included part of the upstairs front bedroom where two children sleep. We were told they were hyperactive and play in their room long after their regular sleep time starts.

Problem: How does a person or family benefitting from a geospiral's Yin energy reduce or turn it off? Unlike geopathic zones which are normally clearly defined and rise in vertical lines above the ground, the geospiral radiates outward (1) with energy rings, and (2) it creates a semi-globe above itself.

If at any time you find any Earth energy annoying or disruptive of one's desire to enjoy a relaxed and normal life, a person can always decree it neutralized or reduced.

Find yourself in a meditative state and say to whoever you pray to: "In the name of the Holy Spirit I decree this energy that is affecting our lives be neutralized or reduced to a safe level. I ask this be performed with love and light. Amen!" Say it just once in a firm, no nonsense voice. Do not repeat. Repetition in prayer is a sign of weakness or a suggestion that Holy Spirit suffers auditory problems. Normally however, geospiral energy is beneficial to one's health and sometimes the best thing is to learn to live with it.

## A GEOSPIRAL COMES VISITING:

The Native Ancestors were and their descendants still are very conscious of both the geospiral forces and the Cosmic connections of spirals. In New Mexico there are many petroglyphs carved or painted on rocks and dowsers will normally find geospirals in the vicinity. Such places were and are sacred to the Native Indians.

During one of our treks in New Mexico, Betty Lou came up with an intriguing supposition. "Is it possible that when humans are gathered together for prayers calling for healing and energy or simply to give thanks to God, they are actually creating or even attracting a geospiral force field?"

It was one of those strange ideas that stayed in our minds until some months later, it happened to us.

Our New Jersey home is situated about a quarter of a mile from the old Quaker/Friends Gathering Place at Arney's Mount. There are several geospirals in the parking lot, in fact when we were doing dowsing workshops, we would normally take participants to the Quaker House.

One evening at one of our weekly meditation and spiritual development circles, I demonstrated an L-rod in the search position with the request: "Show me the nearest geospiral." It usually pointed north towards the Quaker House but this time it was different — it suddenly swung round and pointed south.

Totally surprised we followed the rod into the front garden and discovered not just one but several seven ring geospirals. From a workshop point of view this was very convenient, then a few days later something else occurred, we both had difficulty sleeping. A fast check with the rods showed a geospiral was now centered by Betty Lou's side of the bed. We were forced to lovingly decree it relocated a safe distance away and this happened a day or so later. The others remain in the garden and their energy is both beautiful and relaxing.

This does not answer Betty Lou's original thoughts—do human activities such as meditation and prayer actually trigger or attract earth energies such as geospirals? It is one of those "which came first" situations the chicken or the egg? It would be interesting to discover if this were true. It would open new doors to latent human powers. Personally I believe in the old Universal Cosmic Law of Attraction.

## CHECK YOUR HOME AREA:

One ideal way of gaining experience with geospirals is to conduct a survey of your own immediate environment. In the summer months we hang our hats near the Northern New York villages of Chaumont and Three Mile Bay.

Right in the center of Chaumont is the Copely House. Built as a large family home and office by Alexander Copely in 1852 it is now a community facility and various organizations hold meetings and workshops there. Early in our studies a survey indicated two seven ringed geospirals immediately outside the front windows so any functions inside would be well within the Area of Influence so we were looking forward to attending a dinner there.

Everyone attending seemed very jovial and talkative and a casual observer would have sworn the refreshments were laced with strong stuff. The only liquids served were iced tea, coffee and water.

A lady who regularly attends classes there said: "Oh, it's such a beautiful place. Everyone is so relaxed and happy."

While searching for local geospirals, the rods pointed to a meadow where Black Angus cows often gathered near a rock in the center. The owners were intrigued and asked us to show where the geospiral was. After being chased by a bull in an earlier life, I was hesitant. Anyway, we found the energy exactly where the rod had indicated. The cows simply glanced at us with seemingly glassy eyes as if they might have been on something.

We did a survey of Mount Holly, New Jersey and found various nests of geospirals indicating there had been a strong presence of Native Ancestors.

For instance on the mount in Mount Holly, which is a park populated with great trees, there are at least five geospirals around the summit. The view is nothing to write home about because of the greenery, but it is a great place to hang out and relax as many local residents have found.

Across the nearby High Street and down a block there is the Sacred Heart Church and next door in an older building there is the Chapel of the Blessed Sacrament with a geospiral set in front of the altar. Speaking from personal experiences it is a great place to sit, meditate, relax and talk to Holy Spirit or whoever you pray to.

Which brings back a memory of Santa Fe, New Mexico and the Cathedral Basilica of St. Francis of Assisi Santa Fe where there is a geospiral in the Chapel of the Blessed Sacrament. Again, it's situated in front of the altar.

"There's a lot of energy in this place," I whispered to my old healing guide Chang.

"For people who come here either to pray or attend a service they are subjected to a very powerful healing energy," he said. "You can feel it, yes?"

I nodded an affirmation. "When Bishop Lady and the French architect Antoine Molly built this place they must have been fully aware of what they were doing. They must have felt the power of this geospiral. After all, it covers not only the chapel but also the front of the main church and the altar."

Chang smiled. "Lady would have accepted it as the Hand of God."

"And the old pueblo ancestors, the Indians?"

"The Cathedral Park is situated at the center of the old pueblo and the geospiral is exactly where they had their kiva, their sacred space," he said. "It's a good place for receiving healing both physically and in the mind. It's best to sit and meditate for a while."

When we originally researched the geospiral energies at Los Alamos, New Mexico we were unable to access the Fuller Lodge because it was closed. This was the epicenter of the famous World War II Manhattan Project. Built in 1928 as the remote and elite Ranch School for Boys it served as a dining room and kitchen. The building still stands today as an architectural tribute to the old school.

An interesting phenomenon: the school was renowned for its healthy lifestyle and very few students ever quit. One wonders if the founder, businessman Ashley Pond was aware of the powerful energies resonating at Los Alamos.

The school produced such controversial people as William S. Burroughs, the novelist who wrote *The Naked Lunch*, Gore Vidal who brought homosexuality into the spotlight with *The City and the Pillar* and John Crosby, the American musician who went on to create the Santa Fe Opera was also educated at the school. Ashley Pond's daughter Peggy Pond Church born at Watrous a community on the east side of the Sangre de Cristo Range, became a renowned New Mexican poet and author.

J. Robert Oppenheimer who knew of the place and its energies from his long horse-riding treks in the 1930s, urged the powers in Washington DC to take it over. This they did and during the Manhattan Project it served as a dining room, kitchen and original offices and four geospirals scattered outside may have inspired the work.

It is little wonder the Fuller Lodge complex is now a community building used for art displays, social gatherings and meetings. It houses the Art Center at Fuller Lodge, the Archives and Research Library of the Historical Museum, and the Los Alamos Arts Council. Of course the Los Alamos National Laboratory still operates there under its shroud of secrecy.

We finally achieved access to the Fuller Lodge in 2011 and in the great hall our search rods pointed to the huge fireplace. That is where a 49-ring geospiral radiates, the alpha of the nest, functions in the center of the grate.

Was Oppenheimer aware of the nests of geospirals with their inspiring and motivating energies? Is the Los Alamos Arts Council aware? Did Lady and Molly know what they were doing when they planned and built the Gothic and Romanesque cathedral with its special chapel for prayer — who knows? One is inclined to think it is more than just a coincidence.

The reader will observe throughout this journey in Earth energies that the biographies of people who pioneered places never mention dowsing, divination or even intuitive skills. For instance why did a corporation build a large pyramid on a leyline in downtown Philadelphia? If you watch local television news programs chances are you will see it but no one appears to mention it. We are going to try and find out later.

Back to earth: If dowsers search for geospirals and leys, they will find them, be surprised and enjoy. The motto is: Look and ye shall find. Now, before we leave the mechanics of dowsing, one more important chapter.

# DIGITAL MAP DOWSING

Map dowsing has been a dowsing practice almost as long as cartographers created them. The first maps appear to have been generated by the Sumerians who also came up with the first geographic reference system, the ancestor of today's GPS used on Google Earth and in this book.

Prior to the digital age, dowsers with sharply pointed pendulums would work over high definition charts to find water, oil, minerals, lost objects, remote archaeological sites, various Earth energies and geopathic stress sites. Then came the Digital Age and things started to change.

Today the map-reading dowser can sit in his or her home study and with a laptop equipped with a comfortably sized screen search for any of the Earth energies mentioned above or indeed in this book. The sprawling and cumbersome paper maps have gone and the land is now shown on a computer screen.

The display by Google Earth is a virtual globe, a working map of the world with geographical information. Originally called EarthViewer 3D it was created by Keyhole Inc, a company funded by the Central Intelligence Agency (CIA) and was acquired by Google in 2004.

Using Google Earth dowsers can chart any energy including their favorite water reservoirs, anywhere in the world and using different magnification or enlargement opportunities dowse for water, oil, and energy sources, and of course leys and geospirals. Dowsers can even track the critical Areas of Influence created by leys and nests of geospirals and something we are calling the Cosmic Principle.

It is an incredible and mind-challenging resource. Imagine you can dowse an Eskimo's backyard in the Arctic or check on energy zones crossing the Kremlin Square in Moscow or check some crippled pyramids in the Nubian Desert. It happens.

This facility dawned in our lives a couple of years ago when I happened to check Google Earth for any walking paths near our New Jersey home.

Half a mile away a particular farm with a long driveway off a main road caught my attention I wondered if there were any negative geopathic zones in that area.

One method with laptop dowsing is to hold a pointed instrument over the displayed landscape and holding a pendulum in the right hand ask: "Are there any geopathic zones in this picture?" An old and empty ballpoint pen does nicely as a pointer.

Receiving a positive answer I slowly moved the pointer along the highway and when it reached the farm driveway the pendulum reacted vigorously. Doubting this success, I repeated the experiment. Again positive! Google Earth provided a grid reference which I noted on a blotter. A few minutes later we drove to the farm less than a mile away.

The rods crossed right where the farm driveway intersects the road. Checking the coordinates on Garmin GPS: Spot on! It was exactly as I had recorded on my laptop at home. Over the next few days and weeks we tested the system on leys and nests of geospirals and became generally elated. Then one day a challenge came from afar.

A young engineer named Don who lives with his family in Perth, Western Australia had read on my website about regular dowsing services and now needed help.

"How can I dowse my house for spirits?" he emailed and gave me the address. "It's haunted!"

Google Earth provided an excellent view of the target. The pendulum revealed a negative geopathic zone running across the north-west corner of his place, a bungalow or ranch house with a flatfish roof close to Jackadder Lake.

"You're clear regarding spirits and haunting," I wrote to him. "You do have a geopathic zone. It's a subterranean water vein, twenty feet down, averaging eleven inches wide and running over clay. "

"Would that account for my eight year old son thinking there's a monster or a ghost in the closet?" Don asked.

"Yes, it happens," I said and promptly explained the vein in relation to the home.

"My wife knows a thing or two, she knows how to use a pendulum and confirms what you say," replied Don. "It runs from the closet across the head of his bed."

That day I emailed instructions on how to get steel or bronze plated rods and position them across the vein on both sides of the house. Normally I use 1/8" by 36" rods obtained from a local welding supplies store. Don acquired some and a day or so later emailed me. "The room actually feels clear. It's different. So how did you do that? Are you a blinkin' wizard, mate?"

I told him about Google Earth and the pendulum .

"It's like being across the street," he said with a short laugh.

"Some 11,600 miles away," I replied.

"Do you do this sort of thing often?"

"Enough. I'm sitting in New Jersey Google Earthing the Great Pyramid of Giza in Egypt."

"Really? My wife and I are going there when the lad gets a bit older. Do they have negative energy there?"

"No, just the reverse. There's a massive energy vortex right under the Great Pyramid," I said casually. "When you get to Cairo and the pyramid find a nearby rock, chair or a stretch of desert, sit on it and relax for ten to fifteen minutes. You'll feel something wonderful."

"Yeah? Why?" Now he was cautious.

"It's Yin. Cosmic energy and it is so relaxing you'll be reluctant to leave. Most visitors stand, gape, take pictures and wander around the site. Few pause to relax in the abundant healing energy," I told him. "When you get back home drop me a line."

"Will do, Mister Bob. Will do."

Somehow I did not tell Don I was dowsing the Great Pyramid at Giza for ley lines. It would have taken too long. Besides, it was complicated and as Betty Lou once commented "Some people might think its spooky."

# DOWSING "BLIND" FOR ANCIENT ENERGIES

As in any dowsing operation one must focus on the target which we mentioned earlier. This applies to walking with rods across a field looking for a target, or sitting at a laptop and using a pendulum and pointer. Focus, pure and simple is the essence of effective dowsing. If the dowser has a cluttered mind with a lot of chattering thoughts, learn to relax and focus or find another occupation. A clear mind focused on a target is critical.

Something discovered early on: it is easier to focus on the subject if the eyes watch the pendulum and not the world on a screen. This is called Blind Dowsing because the operator is not looking at the map, in this case the screen. It is quite easy to be distracted when searching for energy centers in the middle of a city, particularly if the place is an exotic location like Rome, Paris or Cairo.

When we search for a ley I use four tools. A pendulum on a short chain of about three inches, the second is a sharp pointer. An old and empty ballpoint pen is good. Third is a writing pad with a wad of pages and fourth is a working pen.

Bring up a large area and ask if there are any leys on the map being displayed. If the answer is affirmative, ask for a number. If the answer is one, the process is simple, give it a pet name and refer to it by that name. If there are two or three leys it is well to refer to them as "Ley One" and "Ley Two," etc.

Let us work with one. The question: Does it run laterally or vertically across this picture (screen)? If it is vertical start moving the pointer slowly across the screen from left to right. If the response is lateral move the pointer from either top to bottom of the screen or vice versa. Perform this task slowly.

If blind dowsing is your forte turn away from the pointer and focus on the pendulum which I have at the side of the laptop. It is here you can repeat the words "Show me the ley," or if you have already established a name use that. The pendulum will swing back and forth until the pointer approaches the ley. Then it speeds up. When it starts to rotate vigorously you need to "feel" the peak of the rotation. The peek dictates when the pointer is on target.

The moment the pointer has passed, the pendulum starts to slow down. Bring the pointer back so the pendulum peaks again. You can now look at the screen and move your mouse to where the pointer is located.

Next, enlarge the map on Google Earth until streets, roads, bridges, buildings, rivers, lakes are clearly in view and refine the search. The pendulum's maximum swing will tell you the exact location, normally within a few feet. Mark it with your mouse, then write down the coordinates seen at the bottom right of the screen.

At this point some bright kid may well accost you with: "How is the pendulum swinging when no one is watching the pointer."

Depending on the questioner you can reply: "It's a magic wand," or if he understands dowsing you might say: "My higher consciousness sees without eyes." The challenge then is to explain higher consciousness.

Now, alternatively, if you wish to dowse direct using your eyes that is fine. There is a caution here. Make sure you dowse without any biases. These can throw a student dowser completely off course. Anyway, back to finding a ley.

The next step is to discover the route of the ley. You can watch the pointer if you wish. Move the pointer around the area until it peaks again perhaps a fair distance away. A mile or so is excellent. As the route is revealed by the pendulum, record the coordinates again.

If they are accurate the numbers will project the ley's route miles, even hundreds of miles because ley energy always appears to travel in straight lines.

If you have a circular contractor, that too will give a more accurate direction of the ley. For instance, Google Earth always indicates a basic North. Keep an alert eye on this indicator, as you enlarge an area because North is shifty and inclined to move silently without telling you.

In summation: Blind Dowsing eliminates human bias and relies completely on Higher Consciousness. You can of course work the fully aware state using a sharply pointed pendulum as the pointer. Many of the readings in this book were done with blind dowsing and a substantial number were confirmed with actual visits.

This technique is a bit "spooky" for some because it does raise the interesting question what or who is watching the pointer move across the screen to enable the pendulum to respond so accurately. Frankly, after conducting hundreds of confirmed readings I fully believe the human higher consciousness is completely aware. How it accomplishes this is something else. The more this technique is practiced the better it seems to function.

This technique is so powerful that the digital dowser can actually plot which side of a city street a leyline exists and at what point it gradually changes sides, without the dowser leaving the office. This occurred in Philadelphia's very long Broad Street as we will write later and also with geospirals at the hub of Spiritualism a few miles east of Lake Erie.

# EARTH ENERGIES AMONG THE SPIRITS

For 136 years people enjoying Spiritualism have been beating the path to a small community called the Lily Dale Assembly in western New York State. The village is on a peninsular jutting out into the three Cassadaga Lakes and comes to life for a few summer months with lecturers and spirit communicators talking, demonstrating and giving messages from loved ones on the Other Side, the Spirit World — Heaven, if you like.

Always curious about the energies there, I browsed Lily Dale with Google Earth and asked for the "nearest ley line." The nearest is a line that flows south-south-east between Buffalo's Jefferson Avenue at High Street and the tiny hamlet of Armor near Hamburg, NY. There was nothing affecting Lily Dale.

However, in answer to the question: "Are there any geospirals within the community?" the pendulum was suddenly driven with a burst of enthusiasm. The target was a location known as "The Stump."

For newcomers the "Inspiration Stump" is a quiet spiritual retreat found at the end of a trail in the Leolyn Woods. Services are held twice a day in the grove at no charge. Since 1898 mediums at The Stump have been giving messages to those in the audience. The Assembly's website adds "you may well renew your own Spiritual energies."

The distance between our laptop in Pemberton, New Jersey to Lily Dale is about 380 miles. Nevertheless in map-dowsing distance is no problem. The pointer and the pendulum together with higher consciousness found a total of seven geospirals in the immediate area behind The Stump. This is opposite to the audience side. The alpha geospiral we dowsed was about seven paces behind the stump projecting an Area of Influence covering the entire Stump site.

After hearing our remote findings, medium Joanne Pfleiderer and her friend and dowser Caroline Jenner visited the site May 6th 2016 and worked independently to confirm each other's reports.

"We located a geospiral center about 20 feet beyond the white picket fence that's in back of The Stump in Lily Dale. We both immediately got a positive reading here when we entered the area and asked the question, "Is this the location of the main geospiral?" We were also able to confirm each other's results," said Joanne.

Signs of geospiral energies are unusual growth patterns in the trees and the two observed this. "Then, we noticed three rings of very old trees in the west-south-west. There are quite unusual circular growth patterns in the forest. We located additional geospirals in each of these tree circles," she said.

Near these trees, there is a marker for the "Healing Tree." The tree is long gone now but, says Joanne, "We felt the healing earth energy was still there."

Before they started surveying The Stump's geospiral energy field they both placed something at the base of the stump, inside the iron fence. Caroline placed a pair of socks and Joanne put a pillow to soak up healing energy.

The next day Lily Dale Board member Neal Rzepkowski went to conduct repairs to the cap as well as the deteriorating iron fence surrounding The Stump when an unusual energy event surprised him.

"As soon as I removed the fence," he says "I felt a rush and swirling of energy which quickly spread over the whole area. It was as if some of the vortex energy of The Stump that had been 'fenced in' and 'capped off' began to move more freely once these were removed."

"Lucky for us, our little objects soaked up some of that grand energy to bring healing to our loved ones back at home," said Ms. Pfleiderer.

# RELAX AS YOU DOWSE

I t does help to get into an altered state of consciousness before using the pendulum or performing any dowsing and divining. One simple and easy way is to close your eyes and pretend to look up into the inside of your forehead for five or ten seconds then open your eyes. This action alone puts a person into a light alpha state which is great for quality dowsing.

It also helps a dowser if he or she spends a few minutes every day in meditation. It raises the intuitive levels and creates a better comfort zone for the higher consciousness.

The how-to instruction is over. It is time to travel to find leys and geospirals.

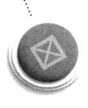

# BOOK TWO

## THE SEARCH FOR PYRAMID POWER

Pyramids have been discovered in many areas of the world and apart from the traditional theory expounded by archaeologists, Egyptologists, New Agers and other gurus, no one has really fathomed the real purpose of these monuments outside of them serving as burial places, or necropolises — cities of the dead for dignitaries large and small. Traditionalists cling to this supposition in spite of the demonstrated fact few pyramids have ever contained relics of the dead.

The Great Pyramid first slipped into my young life while serving in the British Royal Air Force at El Firdan in 1952. A weekend trip to Cairo, resulted in a brief visit to the Giza Plateau. The last existing member of the Seven Wonders of the World with its possible mystic and historical aspects failed to impress so my Air Force colleagues and I stood and gazed for a few fleeting minutes. The old Sphinx appeared more challenging than the stone blocks that seem to tower in the cold light of January. Several took turns in mounting odorous camels which if one was not looking, you became covered in slimy spit. Someone with a Kodak Brownie took pictures, but it all happened so briefly because everyone possessed thirst-driven desires to spend time drinking Stella Beer in an Egyptian bar.

Reflecting back my sensitivities to such things as higher consciousness, Cosmic awareness, energy manifestations and spirit communications were either nonexistent or slumbering in some obscure basement of my mind.

An elderly Arab with a long, drawn face clad in a well worn gallibaya tried to sell me a number of things in this order — watches, two miniature cameras and finally a girl who could not have celebrated a 12th birthday. No one took him seriously, in fact several airmen started joking, an act that made the Arab annoyed to the point of extreme shouting with arms waving.

Suddenly, two uniformed men wearing tarbooshes or fez hats, I know not which, appeared, voiced sharp Arabic commands and chased off the peddler. They then promptly urged our small group of airmen to return to our base in the Suez Canal Zone. It was the eve of the Egyptian Revolution in 1952 when a military coup ousted King Farouk.

Four years later in 1956, now as an award-winning news photographer and journalist, I was back in Cairo covering the political aftermath of the Egyptian takeover of the Suez Canal company. Australia's prime minister Robert Menzies headed negotiations in Cairo with President Gamal Nasser. It was a hectic chase organized by the Egyptian PR people. When two journalists said they planned to visit the Great Pyramid in the late afternoon, I enthusiastically agreed. Ten minutes later, a call from my Cyprus base in Nicosia, urged me to return to the island that very afternoon. So, I missed the opportunity.

The Great Pyramid was so elusive but Egypt was not. In November I was back in the Land of the Pharaohs as an accredited war correspondent covering the Suez War and the Great Pyramid seemed as far off as ever. As if to taunt me, that winter my father in England gave me an antique book entitled *Egypt under the Pharaohs* by Heinrich Brugsch-Bey, the 19th century German Egyptologist who became director of the School of Egyptology in Cairo. Did my father have any thoughts that I would be reading the book sixty years later when writing this one. Life is weird.

My final departure from the Middle East and Egypt was in 1964 and I never did get to witness the insides of the Great Pyramid. When I learned the gentle art of dowsing and its brother, metaphysics, I eventually started a small collection of pyramids — mostly incense burners, but still pyramids. There was something mysterious about the great monument at Giza that attracted me — and I failed to understand why. Eventually I would come to comprehend and appreciate the Cosmic powers of the great pyramid and it started with a double pronged sword — a novel that was partly based on deep human history and partly science fiction.

*UNPLUGGED: The Return of the Fathers* told of ghost pyramids dotted strategically along the Earth's 30th north and south latitudes around the world. The exercise gave me insights into exploring the energies manifested by the ancient pyramids.

Like hundreds, probably thousands of other pyramid explorers I felt drawn to investigate these ancient monuments, not as an archaeologist, which I'm not, but as a dowser seeking energies. As it happened I was not dismayed and the revelations changed my life again.

# THE GREAT PYRAMID AT GIZA

If you have a GPS navigator and risk driving the helter-skelter traffic of Cairo where all drivers are addicted to creating cacophony with their auto horns and head for these coordinates 29° 58′45.06" N 31° 08′03.13" E you will not only get there, your car will actually ram the great monument and someone will get a news story.

Alternatively a thirty minute taxi ride from downtown Cairo will get you in good shape when you arrive at the oldest of the Seven Wonders of the World and the only one to remain vaguely intact even after various earthquakes, human wars and disturbances, plus normal wear and tear from the elements. We are talking about the Great Pyramid of Giza.

The traditionalists will tell you the Great Pyramid was built around 2,600 BCE during the reign of Pharaoh Khufu a.k.a. Cheops. Next to the Great Pyramid stand two others. The slightly smaller one is attributed to

Cheop's son and successor Kephren. The other, still smaller, is attributed to Kephren's successor, the grandson of Cheops, Mykerionos. To the south-east of the Great Pyramid lies the Sphinx like a worn out dog basking in Eternity.

The Great Pyramid of Giza is the world's largest single stone building in human history and was built to stand the passing of time. Many Egyptologists and others still cling to the idea it was built as a tomb, a preservation center, around 2560 BCE during the fourth dynasty of Pharaoh Khufu.

This is based on a mark discovered in an interior chamber that claimed to name the work gang and made reference to Khufu. This mark may be fraudulent as the Great Pyramid contains no other markings of any sort.

One school of radical thinking suggests the monument was created as a navigation beacon for an ancient civilization that colonized Earth in the time prior to accepted human history. The colonizers, according to ancient Sumerian clay tablets, genetically engineered and bred humanity as we know it. Thus the Giza pyramid served as a guiding instrument and probably more. Some sources including this author are inclined to believe it was built according to a simple Cosmic formula active thousands of years ago — and is still active today! But there is more, infinitely much more to the Great Pyramid in terms of dowsing its energy as we will see.

The size of the Great Pyramid dazzles the mind. For a start it covers 13 acres and its volume or mass is 90 million cubic feet. It contains an estimated 2.3 million pieces of gray limestone each measuring three feet thick and weighing an average of 2.5 tons a piece. Its four sides are perfectly shaped, each measuring 756 feet across the base. From the bottom it sweeps up to a height of 481 feet and it is so designed and positioned that the sun shines on all four sides at once.

Back in history the sides were originally layered with white limestone blocks each weighing about 15 tons, immaculately finished and each set at an angle so that the rise would be 52 degrees from horizontal. The finish, the joints between the blocks, was so precise and so perfect that a human hair would not fit between the cracks.

The construction cement was extremely fine and strong. Where did it originate. So far, its origin has defied analysis. Incidentally, the white limestone has mostly gone, carted off to build Cairo.

The total mass of the Great Pyramid is calculated to be 93 million cubic feet with a weight of approximately seven million tons.

For its size, the Great Pyramid contains a minimum of available space. Apart from three main passages which lead to three chambers or rooms, there is nothing else. From top to bottom they are the King's Chamber, the Queen's Chamber and the Subterranean Chamber.

Made out of granite, the King's Chamber measures about 34 feet by 17 feet and is about 19 feet high. It also contains what experts believe is a granite coffin. It should be noted that all the passages in the Great Pyramid are all in the same vertical plane.

Almost vertically underneath is the so-called Queen's Chamber. Granite is absent and the room has a rough floor and a gabled limestone roof. The ancient walls are mysteriously encrusted with salt sometimes as much as ½ inch thick. Chamber dimensions are 18 feet 10 inches by 17 feet 2 inches. It has a double pitched ceiling at its highest point, formed by huge blocks of limestone.

The name Queen's Chamber is a misnomer. The custom among Arabs was to place their women in tombs with gabled ceilings (as opposed to flat ones for men), so this room came to be labeled by the Arabs as the Queen's Chamber.

In the middle of the north side there exists a passage, three feet wide, four feet high that leads down into a Subterranean Chamber surrounded by solid rock. It is 100 feet below ground level and is positioned exactly 600 feet under the apex point. Thus all Chamber complexes are within vertical alignment of the apex point — an important aspect as we shall see when we discuss Cosmic energy.

It was copied by other Egyptian rulers to the extent the country has between 118 and 138 pyramids.

Egyptologists and other experts have generally agreed that the Egyptian pyramids were built as tombs for the country's pharaohs and their consorts during the Old and Middle Kingdom periods. Most archaeologists suggest they are all inferior to the Great Pyramid. In fact the Philadelphia Theologian and Pyramidologist Joseph A. Seiss in 1877 described them as "blind and bungling imitations of the Great Pyramid."

Over the past two centuries many notable people — historians, archaeologists, architects, engineers, physicists, mathematicians, writers and others have tried to figure reasons why it was built on the Giza plateau which is, as deserts usually are, very arid.

For dowsers the answer is simple. The Great Pyramid is not only an Earth energy center, it also attracts Cosmic energy, even though the pyramid itself is crippled as we shall see. Crippled? Oh, yes, definitely.

## COPYING? CANNOT BE DONE

The common idea is the Egyptian hierarchy used countless thousands of workers and slaves to chisel and move blocks of rock weighing from two to 200 tons each. Construction specialists frequently theorize the Egyptians were forced to use primitive log rollers, ropes, pulleys and manpower not only to transport the blocks of stone across the River Nile but to hoist them into place hundreds of feet up.

It has been well demonstrated that these basic ideas did not work then and they do not work in recent times.

In 1978 a Japanese research group funded by Nissan acquired permission from the Egyptian Department of Antiquities to build a small model of the Great Pyramid, 60 feet in height. Like the ancient Egyptians the workers would use only primitive tools.

The project struck hard reality when the team, armed with hammers and chisels went to a nearby limestone quarry and attempted to cut the stone. The task force eventually resorted to modern pneumatic hammers to remove the stone. One hundred men were employed to move each one across the desert sand and the Nile but in the end the team was forced to use trucks and river barges. To tackle the actual building of this small pyramid, cranes and even a helicopter were used to place the rocks into position.

When the model pyramid was completed it was nowhere near the perfection of the Great Pyramid where stones were laid so accurately, it is difficult to pass a knife blade through the cracks.

The Nissan funded project clearly showed that many academics are stuck in a rut if they believe the Great Pyramid was constructed by human energy using primitive methods. And yet, that is the dominant teaching in world universities and schools along with academics working in the field. They were and are taught this way, they believe the teachings are true and are forced to tread the narrow path that fails to permit radical thinking or theories. The bottom line clearly shows that the true builders of the Great Pyramid at Giza were forces from another realm, another culture that possessed capable technology. There are also energies at Giza which many people ignore, except dowsers. Our journey continues.

# TRACKING DOWN THE BUILDERS

Back in 1849, the British Archaeologist, Austin Henry Layard discovered 22,000 clay tablets in the Ancient Sumerian city of Nineveh on the banks of the Tigris River in an area now known as Iraq. Carved in cuneiform script on soft clay it is one of the earliest known writing systems, created by the Sumerians some 6,000 or more years ago.

Author, researcher and Cuneiform translator, Zecharia Sitchin spent more than 30 years deciphering some of the Sumerian Tablets. In his 1976 book *The 12th Planet* Sitchin claims the Sumerian text describes an alien race named the "Anunnaki" who came to Earth from an undiscovered planet in our Solar System, beyond Neptune called Nibiru.

Strangely, the ancient tablets also contain drawings showing the planets Neptune, Uranus and Pluto, among other astral bodies revolving around the Sun. Modern day astronomers maintain that Neptune was not discovered by stargazers until 1846. William Herschel discovered Uranus, initially named George's Star after King George III, in 1781 while Pluto was not discovered until 1930.

In 1514 the Polish astronomer Nicolaus Copernicus talked about the planets revolving around the Sun but it was not until he died in 1543 that the book containing his observations was published. It took almost 100 years for his work to take hold. That's when Galileo Galilei in 1632, building on Copernicus' work, claimed that the Earth orbited the sun. He promptly found himself under house arrest for committing heresy against the Catholic church.

One major discovery in the old Sumerian clay tablets concerns the Creation story. Written in Sumeria 1,000 years before the Jewish Captivity in Babylon, it was adopted and names were modified by the Jews and thus became the Torah — also known as the first five chapters of the Old Testament.

Many translators of Cuneiform tablets glibly branded all the Sumerian tablet stories as "myths," seemingly without thinking things through and perhaps, fearing angry reactions from the masses attending mainline churches.

The more one works to understand the Sumerian tablets, the more feasible it becomes that space travelers from another planet or star system visited Earth and gave the Sumerians a leading edge in the evolutionary mind for great techniques and modalities.

Zacharia Sitchin maintained that the Giza pyramids were built by space travelers and Earth colonizers called the Anunnaki. It formed a critical point in the Landing Corridor that served the post-Diluvial Spaceport in the Sinai on the 30th parallel, no less.

That's another fascinating aspect of the Great Pyramid. The real builders of the Great Pyramid of Giza knew that Planet Earth was in fact spherical. Not only that, they mapped a grid reference system with both latitudes and longitudes for global navigation purposes. The construction of the Great Pyramid took place a short distance south of latitude 30 degrees and 30 degrees longitude. In fact the latitude point is about a two minute drive north towards Cairo.

The Egyptians, the Assyrians, the Sumerians were not the Stone Age brigades our historians would have us believe. According to the old clay tablets the Sumerians invented mathematics and through this developed a system of numbers based on units of 60. Called the sexagesimal system

46

it now forms the basis for measuring time, angles and geographic coordinates. Time is still measured at 60 seconds in a minute, 60 minutes in an hour and the division of a circle contains 360 degrees. Remember, 360 reduces to the Cosmic Nine.

Invented is perhaps the wrong word. It is highly possible the Sumerians were taught many valuable techniques that have been handed down over the generations.

The Sumerians are credited with building the first cities, the first libraries. They instituted the first monarchies with a priest-king who exercised divine authority — hence organized religion. They developed organized agricultural lands, provided complex irrigation systems and trading systems. First in pictographs and then in writing, they developed a written communications system called cuneiform through which came the first books — literature! That gave rise to The Epic of Gilgamesh which tells of a Sumerian king undertaking a long and perilous journey to discover the secret of eternal life. The priests observed the skies and created calendars based on what they saw. From this came 12 lunar months with leap years to catch up with the Sun's year. From this emerged astronomy.

For instance, today's Jewish calendar 5776 (2016 in the Gregorian calendar) dates back to Sumerian and Babylonian history and the lives of Adam and Eve.

This was not all. The Sumerians developed the wheel which allowed for the movement of trade goods and people. The Assyrians eventually adopted it to move large armies across the Middle East.

How is it that a civilization — the Sumerian– was able to develop so many significant attributes, systems that still influence and form important parts of our lives today? Our GPS — Global Positioning System such as Garmin, TomTom and Google Earth — use the legacies of the Sumerian civilization. As various translators of the Sumerian tablets have shown all or most of these developments were gifts, brought to Earth by space travelers known as the Anunnaki colonists.

In December 2015, the University of Vermont reported in a study that a 300-million-year natural pattern on Earth ended 6,000 years ago "because of human activity." Should not that be "Sumerian activity" or even "Anunnaki activity"? Some authorities suggest this was the real time for the start of building pyramids world wide.

But here in Egypt there is more inside the Great Pyramid that suggests Cosmic origins. Deep in the heart of the monument is the granite King's Chamber which is so surrounded by masonry that the temperature of this inner sanctum maintains an almost even 68 degrees Fahrenheit. This is in addition to the fact it is furnished with a system of ventilating tubes to maintain a normal living condition.

Consider what incredible mind figured 68 degrees? This is exactly midway between freezing and the boiling points of water. It is also the recommended temperature for most homes and offices to maintain comfortable living and working conditions for human habitation.

This poses the question: Why? Most Earth people interested in the Great Pyramid admit they have no idea why the chamber was created to provide natural living conditions in this or any other age. Perhaps one day an intelligence out in space will take credit for the design, provide answers and satisfy human curiosity.

But wait, there is another mystery. The sides of the Great Pyramid face directly north, south, east and west, which means the builders of the monument knew the locations of the north and south poles. Why was it necessary to build the great monument exactly half way between the north pole and the equator with such mathematical precision?

There is another intriguing aspect of the Great Pyramid suggesting Cosmic origins. American Theologian and Lutheran Minister Joseph Augustus Seiss known for his studies in pyramidology notes the vertical height of the Great Pyramid at Giza is 481 feet tall, exactly 1/1,000,000,000 the distance the earth is from the sun. This presents another question: Was it just coincidence, like many other points about the Great Pyramid or was it that the pyramid was required to be a specific distance from the sun to operate correctly? Again, this is another of the seemingly endless questions.

We humans with our insatiable hunter-conqueror egos often get bent out of shape when it is suggested the Great Pyramid was designed and built by any force other than countless thousands of Egyptians sweating and agonizing in the sun for twenty or more years. For that matter most people do not wish to even consider that a force of space travelers colonized Planet Earth for many thousands of years and flew around the continents with greater ease that most people do today. But that is the story written on thousands of clay tablets from Sumeria, now Iraq, which rest in major universities and museums around the world.

The Great Pyramid of Giza is not just a work of Cosmic Art that has been and still is beyond the reach of the human mind and earthly technology. It was and indeed is a sacred point in the Cosmic order of things. When we started studying the energies surrounding the Great Pyramid we had no idea what would surface. When it happened, it was so small and almost insignificant and one wonders why the great explorers in history did not catch onto it.

## THE NEVER ENDING SEARCH FOR ANSWERS

So what is it about the magnetism of the Great Pyramid that attracts at least 14 million visitors annually? Historically the energies have attracted many famous figures, not all innocent tourists. Abdullah al-Mamun who lived about 800 AD was the seventh caliph, ruler of the Islamic Empire of the Abbasid dynasty. A pensive fellow he advocated the study of Greek philosophy and investigated the Great Pyramid at Giza.

Arriving with a small army and unable to find an entrance, his men attempted to break into the walls by boring through the limestone with crude totally unsuitable tools. Many frustrating months passed before they succeeded in gaining entry and once inside they discovered the descending passage.

Eventually they reached the two chambers of the so-called King and Queen and found almost nothing — except an empty red granite box which experts eventually named "The empty coffin." There were no mummies nor human relics and sad to say, no treasure. For al-Mamun the work was a total disappointment.

However, if the mighty caliph had paused to tap the "coffin" he would have heard interesting sounds. As later adventurers would discover it produces sounds like a beautiful singing bowl. One wonders why anyone ever called it a coffin.

In 1637 an English mathematician, astronomer and antiquary John Greaves visited Giza and wrote the first book entitled *Pyramidographia: A Discourse of the Pyramids in Egypt.* The book prompted a stream of international visitors to view and study the phenomenon at Giza.

One French antiquary, Jesuit Pere Claude Sicard, spent 20 years in the first part of the 18th century documenting 20 of the major Egyptian pyramids, two dozen complete temples and over 50 decorated tombs. Sicard visited the Great Pyramid in 1715 and part of his account focused on the unique feature of the empty coffin in the King's chamber. He wrote: "It is formed out of a single block of granite, has no cover and when struck sounds like a bell".

Other visitors, intrigued by the singing coffin noted that the red granite piece is totally devoid of any description. Leading personalities drawn to Giza by this mysterious and beautiful energy included English diplomat Nathaniel Davison who discovered a space in the Great Pyramid, known as "Davison's Chamber" or the "first relieving chamber"; Lord Horatio Nelson who died at the Battle of Trafalgar; Irish-English soldier and statesman Arthur Wellesley, the Duke of Wellington who defeated Napoleon; Lady Ann Arbuthnot; and Brigadier-General Patrick Campbell, military leader, diplomat and amateur archaeologist who served in Egypt. Campbell's Chamber in the Great Pyramid was named in his honor by the discoverer.

Two other people who are said to have spent time alone in the King's Chamber are Alexander the Great and Napoleon Bonaparte. Historians say it is highly possible but difficult to prove with either one.

Various authorities are still at loggerheads over Napoleon who it is claimed while spending time alone in the Great Pyramid, experienced a vision of a spirit, possibly a pharaoh, or as this author suggests, one of the Anunnaki gods. Who knows?

British archaeologist and Egyptologist Sir William Flinders Petrie described the Great Pyramid as "the greatest and most accurate structure the world has ever seen."

In 1932 Edgar Cayce known to many as the "sleeping proph formed readings on the Great Pyramid and placed the construction of it between 10,490 to 10,390 BCE — that's over 7,000 years more than traditional Egyptologists.

Physical explorers are one element, mystical explorers are another.

Over the centuries secret mystery schools have visited and gathered in the vicinity of the Great Pyramid, fully aware that the edifice was not a large burial monument or sarcophagus for a dead pharaoh, but something more Cosmic, perhaps a multi-dimensional channel or a stargate for initiation and transformation. It is a pity they did not use a dowser's pendulum, they would have been astounded. Sometimes people get too close to the physical to experience the Cosmic values.

In recent history musicians Paul Horn and Steven Halpern both performed there. Mr. Halpern says he first visited Egypt in 1980 and maintained it was "a life changing event." The following year, accompanied by his recording engineer he returned to the Great Pyramid and on three separate occasions was granted unprecedented private access.

The result, he says, is a one-of-a kind recording that transports you inside the majestic Kings' Chamber on the magic carpet of sound. "As I tuned in to the energy of ancient ceremonies, sacred chants began to channel through me. Using state-of-the-art recording equipment, the higher harmonics and deeply reverberating acoustic properties of the room were captured on tape." The CD is entitled: *INITIATION: Inside the Great Pyramid.*

# LEYS AND GEOSPIRALS: ATTRACTORS!

The Great Pyramid attracts millions of people every year. Why? Perhaps the mystique of the many stories about the place, perhaps because it is the "place to go" because so many historic figures have trodden its path, or perhaps the energies manifested by leys and geospirals are so powerfully attractive.

If as a dowser you decide to visit the ancient land of the Pharaohs you will quickly find that Egypt has a multiplicity of ley lines and geospirals at various locations. Alexandria, Luxor, Cairo, but the greatest concentration is at the Great Pyramid.

In addition to the leys converging and passing through there are several blind springs in and around the Giza pyramids silently giving off continuous showers of beneficial Yin energy.

This concentration assists the Giza Plateau in ranking as a major vortex along with such sacred places as Glastonbury in England, Mount Ararat in Turkey, Sedona in Arizona, Teotihuacán the Aztecs' City of the Gods in Mexico and Machu Picchu high in the Peruvian Andes. These places with their various attractions all have one thing in common: ley lines.

Each ley produces a force usually of a yin nature, which means it is beautiful, passive, relaxing, inspiring and feminine, all points we discussed earlier. Plus, if you are so inclined you can walk along them in open spaces.

The Great Pyramid at Giza is a gathering point for four leys and they intensify its latent and Cosmic energy. Whatever great mind conceived and built the great monument knew exactly what they were doing from global and Cosmic energy points of view. The ancient pyramid builders did not create a vortex in Egypt, they simply recognized it as a major energy crossroads, enjoyed the energy and used it to their own ends. Humans are naturally drawn to high energy centers much like inhabitants of Nature are always drawn to light.

Right now, as dowsers, let us follow the energy.

# LEYS — THE OLD AND ANCIENT TRACKS

At least four major leys cross the nine acres covered by the Great Pyramid at Giza. Each one generates or radiates an added attractive energy. The ancient trackways have been used by explorers, merchant traders in camel caravans, conquerors and armies, plus millions of ordinary travelers seeking new routes, new places, healing spas and more.

# THE ARARAT -BAALBEK-GIZA- BAHARIYYA LEY.

Distance: 1,850 miles

This north-east to south-west triple-haired ley comes out of the famous snowcapped Mount Ararat in Turkey where Noah's Ark is supposed to have come to rest after the Deluge. It passes through ancient Baalbek in Lebanon which stands about 50 miles from Beirut. Known as Heliopolis or City of the Sun in Roman times Baalbek was considered the holiest of the holy in pagan times because the Temple of Baal or Jupiter existed there. The Romans were fully aware of its energies because they left massive and elegant stoneworks and columns there. But the Roman monument is minuscule by comparison to the megaliths on which they were built.

Massive stones weighing 1,500 tons and measuring 68 x 14 x 14 feet were used in creating the foundations. Archaeologists claim they are the largest worked stones on earth and for most people their origin is a mystery.

Zecharia Sitchin says Sumerian Cuneiform records indicate it was a "landing place of the gods" used by the Anunnaki following recovery from the Deluge.

The ley then runs across Lebanon, the eastern Mediterranean, then to Egypt and to Cairo where it passes through the famous Tahrir Square, then on to the Great Pyramid at Giza. The ley then heads out into Egypt's Western Desert and passes through Bahariyya an oasis town about 225 miles south-west of Giza and Cairo. The oasis which is home to some 30,000 people has at least 14 geospirals close to the ley and probably more throughout the cluster of townships. The area contains many springs, some thermal, such as Ain Bishmu which dates back to Roman times. The oasis towns produce wine, olive oils, dates, and cereals and some travelers call it "Heaven" and now you may understand why. Others have chosen to be buried there. It is at the Bahariyya Oasis you will find an archaeological hotspot — the Valley of the Golden Mummies.

Discovered as late as 1996 it is the largest of its kind. The four-mile strip of desert holds between 5,000 and 10,000 mummies. These bodies of bygone ages are covered with thin layers of gold and wear gypsum masks. Fabulous gilded death masks reflect lifelike faces of real people, rather than the old stereotyped images.

The Egyptian Director of the Department of Antiquities, Dr. Zahi Hawaas says: "These mummies, many sumptuously decorated with religious scenes, represent the very best of Roman-Period mummies ever found in Egypt. These ancient remains are around 2000 years old, but they have withstood the test of time remarkably well."

The actual cemetery area is about four miles from downtown El Bawati and covers about four square miles. This powerful triple-haired ley then continues south-west into the depths of the Great Sahara Desert.

## THE ALEXANDRIA TRIO

Alexander the Great or his personal dowsers must have been well aware of the energy lines along Egypt's Mediterranean Coast because the military leader established the city of Alexandria there. At various points in its colorful and frequently hectic existence it was the capital of Egypt, it became a hotbed of early Christian fathers, the Great Royal Library, considered to be one of the greatest collections in the world, burned down in 48 BCE. The Arabs conquered it, Napoleon visited the area with his French Troops and was later defeated there. All three of the so-called "Cleopatra Needles" — obelisks were shipped from here to London, New York and Paris. In addition author Lawrence Durrell lived in the city and later wrote the famous Alexandria Quartet.

Some might say truly amazing for a place that started as a small fishing center. However, there are at least three leys passing through the metro area today, all attracting millions of sun worshipers, curiosity seekers, photographers, writers and holiday-makers each year.

# ABU QIR — GREAT PYRAMID — PORT SAFAGA LEY

Distance: 434 miles

Abu Qir is a village within Metro Alexandria. It's on a headland or peninsula overlooking the Mediterranean. Right where the ley starts to come out of the sea, under about 30 feet of water and buried in sand, French archaeologists recently discovered the sunken city of Herakleion, the precursor to the once-powerful capital of Alexandria. Underwater visitors frequently compare it to the lost city of Atlantis because huge statues and buildings grace the sandy seabed.

The ley heads south and passes through the Great Pyramid at Giza before flanking the Red Sea and finally breaking from land at Port Safaga. This place was once a great military station for Roman soldiers because of its health spas. Today visitors come to explore the reefs, wander the beaches of black and gold sand dunes or take a day trip to Mons Claudianus to view remnants of the Roman Empire.

# THE EL-AGAMY / GREAT PYRAMID / MOUNT SINAI LEY

Distance known is 430 miles

Another leyline comes out of the Mediterranean a few miles west of the historic Egyptian city of Alexandria and heads south-east to cross the Great Pyramid at the center point. It follows much of the Alexandria-Cairo highway.

After Giza the line continues its course and passes through another sacred spot on Mother Earth — Mount Sinai also known as Mount Horeb on the Sinai Peninsula. The Old Testament records that it was here Moses received from God the Tablets of the Law otherwise known as the Ten Commandments.

The entire area is sacred to three world religions: Christianity, Islam, and Judaism. The mountain is known and revered by Muslims as Jebel

Musa — the Mountain of Moses and Biblical history notes that Abraham was the father of all three religions.

Saddled on the ley is the Orthodox Monastery of St. Catherine. Founded in the 6th century, it is the oldest Christian monastery still in use for its initial function. In addition to the attraction of leys and geospirals, the ancient walls and buildings are of great significance for studies in Byzantine architecture plus the monastery contains outstanding collections of early Christian manuscripts and icons. The rugged mountainous landscape, containing numerous archaeological and religious sites and monuments, forms a perfect backdrop to the ancient place.

As one studies leys and geospirals it becomes quite apparent that these earthly energies have played key roles in the development of great communities both in the distant past and in our recent history.

# THE GREAT NILE LEY: ROSETTA / GREAT PYRAMID / LUXOR

Distance: 543 miles

This is a major triple-haired ley that comes out of the Mediterranean at a village named Rashid, 38 miles east of Alexandria on the International Coastal Road. It's a dusty place but loaded with history of times gone by. Rashid is also called Rosetta after the famous stone discovered in the desert by one of Napoleon's soldiers. The stone with its carvings became a Universal treasure, a gift of the gods, say some, because it was written in three languages: 1. Hieroglyphic used for important or religious documents; 2. Demotic the common script of Egypt; and 3. Greek the common language of the rulers of Egypt. That one stone established modern day communications with ancient writers in deep history.

From Rosetta and heading almost due south, the ley passes through the west side of Cairo, through the center-piece of the Great Pyramid, then heads on almost paralleling the River Nile to the City of Luxor, 400 miles south. There it passes through the Mortuary Temple of Seti 1 on the road to the Valley of the Kings, before crossing the Nile to the east side to pass through the Temple of Karnak.

All these Egyptian leys have been in existence for thousands of years and the fact they are still in existence today shows they are permanent fixtures in the history of Planet Earth. So one wonders just how ancient the leys really are and why do they exist in Nature at all? Why do they run in straight lines which seems contrary to Nature's basic design in spirals? Always more questions.

"They are rivers of life." It was a voice from the Other Side, the Spirit World and it was loud and clear.

For once, I let it stand. No reply. No questions. Something deep inside was hinting a radial change in how we see things. Perhaps some force in the Cosmos was about to produce some answers. Earth energy — leys and geospirals — are one thing, but there is something else. Some strange phenomenon far from old Egypt but everything to do with the Great Pyramid of Giza was about to surface.

# A VOICE FROM THE OTHER SIDE

It happened one evening in the fall of 2014. Betty Lou was preparing supper and I was sitting quietly at the marble breakfast counter and pondering over a small silvery metal pyramid. Purchased recently on the web, it was a nifty incense burner standing just over two inches tall that was destined to sit in my office. Little did I know it would trigger a search for similar mini-pyramids. But right now it was sitting quietly next to the salt and pepper shakers.

Suddenly it changed dimensions and talked. At least, I heard a voice that seemed to hang over the pyramid. Having heard ethereal voices many times I concluded the voice originated in the Spirit World, the Other Side as we mystics refer to it. But today this voice was strangely different.

"Imagination," I thought.

"Go on, test it!" The voice was now loud and clear. A refined English voice the like of which was found at Oxford in the old days.

"Go on, test it," urged the voice, gritty and impatient.

"Test what?

"The pyramid. The one on your breakfast counter."

"Test it for what? And how?"

"Pendulum!" said the voice. "You are excruciatingly slow, Egby. Use your pendulum."

Moments later I retrieved a pendulum from the office, cleared a place on the marble counter and hesitatingly held it over the small silvery pyramid.

As explained in the Dowsing Instruction earlier a pendulum can answer a question in four ways — Yes, No, Cannot Say and Don't Know. My Yes is a swing clockwise, my No is a swing counter-clockwise.

Nothing happened. I gave the pendulum a small push to make it swing clockwise. It was reluctant to move.

Reluctant? How could that be? Pendulums can swing anyway they choose, at least that is the way I had been taught. But my old tried-and-true pendulum was definitely and emphatically reluctant to swing clockwise. More important, I could feel its growing reluctance to swing clockwise.

Then something weird happened.

The glass pendulum started swinging counter-clockwise. Slowly at first then gaining force and swinging faster and faster as if being chased by some invisible hounds. Now totally fascinated and desperate to hold onto the chain, my free left hand grasped my right wrist to steady the hold. The pendulum was now hurtling round at such a speed and force that I feared it would break the little chain and become a glass bullet.

Reluctantly, I broke off and stopped the process. .

Unable to believe what had happened, I ran to my office and used the pendulum on several other pyramids — wooden, sandstone and crystal. The responses were all identical. Initially a hesitancy to swing clockwise, then a definite swing counter-clockwise with a pronounced desire to swing faster and faster. It was all totally surprising and very strange.

Both Betty Lou and her son Ken branded it "spooky."

Over the next little while we accumulated different pyramids — all with the same result. Then a friend found a three-sided pyramid. The pendulum failed to acknowledge it.

"It has to be a four-sided pyramid to get this reaction," I said to Betty Lou. "Pyramids with four sides have a certain power. Pyramids with three or five sides fail. Is it Cosmic?"

"Ask your spirit guides," she suggested. "Where is the voice that started this?"

I recalled the voice. Very British, clear as a bell. Just thinking about a spirit triggers a reaction. Suddenly it was back.

"So what does this mean?" I asked.

"Everything in the Universe is available for the enquiring mind."

"Oh, really? One must have an object, a target upon which the mind may base its inquiries?" I responded.

"We are chippy today, aren't we, young fellow?" came the voice easily. "Why don't you obtain a picture of the Great Pyramid at Giza and test that with your instrument."

Moments later an encyclopedia showed a landscape view of the Great Pyramid flanked by the minor pyramids and the Sphinx. No reaction. The pendulum swung limply back and forth with nowhere to go.

"You need to view the pyramid from the top," urged the voice quietly.

"Who on earth takes a picture of the Great Pyramid from above?"

For some moments I pondered the problem. Then it struck: "Google Earth!"

Moments later I typed "Great Pyramid at Giza" into the search box and the picture on my laptop zoomed in towards the great monument. I adjusted it until my view was looking straight down. Excited, perhaps nervous, I reached for my pendulum and held it over the screen. It seemed impossible that it would demonstrate the strange energy we had found on the mini-pyramids

For a moment the pendulum hovered above the Great Pyramid then as if giving acknowledgment to going clockwise, it suddenly started swinging counter-clockwise. First of all a steady and decisive swing, then as if motivated by a different and enthusiastic power it started going faster and faster. Again I had to hold my wrist to steady the pull. Finally I broke the swinging and stopped the pendulum.

"Pyramid Power!" I muttered exuberantly.

"Cosmic!" said the voice softly as if correcting.

The words seemed strange. Impossible. Why should a photograph taken from way out in space convey or reflect whatever strange power was contained or being manifested by a four-sided pyramid.

And why counter-clockwise? That is one of the glaring and infuriating things about pyramids and the Cosmos. Discover something and it immediately triggers more questions.

First of all, Canadians and Americans use the word to describe the hands of a clock going in reverse. British people use the term anti-clockwise, Americans say counter-clockwise. In dowsing we will use both.

There is another term *sinistral* which means on the left. Most gastropodic shells run clockwise except a sinistral. Strange! That was something I learned from my lifelong buddy and Conchologist S. Peter Dance when we were in Egypt. Also, a sinistral flatfish lies with the left eye uppermost.

What else runs counter-clockwise? From my dowsing lectures I recalled that if you hold a pendulum over a man's head it will swing clockwise but if it is held over a woman's head it swings counter-clockwise.

Does this mean our bodies are all male or all female? Absolutely not. Hold a pendulum over a thumb and watch it swing, then move it over an index finger and it will change direction. Clockwise and counter-clockwise. Male and female. Each of the fingers has a different energy to the one next to it.

So where does all this place pyramid energy?

According to the Taoist gurus everything in Nature and indeed the Cosmos is based on Yin and Yang. It is the mystical concept that calls for balance in our lives. Too much of either side creates an imbalance which prompts suffering and ultimately chaos and destruction. For instance, if a person seized by a desire to live a totally spiritually devoted life becomes cloistered in a monasterial-like home and lives only for prayers to God, it creates an unhealthy Yin imbalance. In Taoism the wheel of life becomes lopsided, impractical and fails to work.

The answer is to get out into the sunshine, breathe the oxygen of the forests and gardens, swim, exercise, climb mountains, work to see the physical beauty of life as created by the Cosmos. See the sunshine. This brings the balance of Yin and Yang within.

So a pyramid generates Yin energy which is passive, intuitive, right-brain creative, compassionate, mystical and healing.

Does pyramid energy heal? And if so, why do small models of pyramids — manufactured of stone, wood, glass or crystal — demonstrate the feminine counter-clockwise energy?

Let us find out.

# TRACKING DOWN PYRAMID POWER

The original and intriguing demonstration at the breakfast counter triggered months of exploring mini-pyramid energy. It matters not how big or small the pyramid is, the pendulum always swings counter-clockwise with a gathering force that makes it difficult to control. We experimented with wood, metal, crystal and soapstone pyramids — the results were always the same.

We even placed the silver metal pyramid on the ground and stood on a small step-ladder with the pendulum directly above. The pendulum swung counter-clockwise. The whole thing failed to make sense.

Then the voice returned: "Have you tried underneath the pyramid?"

It was almost as if we were being led and some spirits were having fun doing it. Betty Lou always claims spirits move things around the house just to tease us.

Underneath? We placed a pyramid on the table and knelt down on the floor and held a pendulum directly below. The result a counter-clockwise spin with a vengeance.

This now raised the question — which way is the energy traveling? Perhaps it is just a column of energy that passes up and down alternating like AC electricity.

These were early days in our studies. Students at our metaphysical development circle found mini-pyramids fascinating and all used their own pendulums with the same results.

"If it's Yin it must be healing energy?" asked one.

At the time I was having a gout attack on my right knee, something I have not had for 50 years. Placing the metal pyramid over my afflicted joint, the discomfort immediately eased. One circle member Mark, suffering arthritis, placed it on his leg and within a few seconds there was an immediate reduction in discomfort.

Amid a chorus of comments there came a logical question: "How does one hold a pyramid over one's pain, even while resting in bed or on the couch?" Michelle suggested strapping a pyramid with bandages over an affliction. The consensus emerged that the idea was good but impractical.

This prompted the question: Do pyramids only work vertically? A large wooden pyramid was placed on its side, supported by a small glass tube. A pendulum was held a short distance away from the point — again counter-clockwise! This meant that the energy generated or attracted by the pendulum is not necessarily vertical, in fact it can and does travel according to where the pyramid apex is pointing.

This experiment jarred the conception that all cosmic energy travels directly up or down. Pyramid energy travels according to whatever direction the apex is pointing.

As research continued this whole assumption was proved incorrect with the discovery of something called Area of Influence. For now we were to believe the pyramid apex was like a gun barrel, shooting out energy. How wrong we were.

This development prompted some deep thought and while pondering I returned to the laptop and Google Earth's high definition view looking straight down on the Great Pyramid at Giza.

What is your secret? So many great minds have pursued your purpose. You have been measured, angled, and reproduced only to trigger theories and more theories. But pendulum reaction to a pyramid was not a theory. It was a fact that anybody, absolutely anybody could demonstrate that a pyramid, big or small was imbued with a power that insisted a pendulum swing counter-clockwise.

"Pendulum," said the voice suddenly.

Wait, at this point it was necessary for me to identify the voice no matter how interesting the suggestions might be.

"Pendulum!" It was blunt and almost as if he might be in a hurry.

I raised a hand. "I have an age-old policy of talking only to disembodied spirits who have names. What's yours?"

"Bernard."

"Plain and simple Bernard? You don't have a sophisticated Greek or Roman name like Zenon, Ra, Gabriel...?"

"Out of my league, actually," said the voice. "Also I am not just plain and simple. I am Bernard."

I could feel the rebuke. "Sorry for being judgmental. It was a slip of the tongue."

"Forgiven," he said. "Now, pendulum."

"We have done that already," I protested softly not wishing to disrupt the calm.

"Pendulum!"

I held one over the digital image of the Great Pyramid. Sure enough, it started swinging counter-clockwise, delivering a hefty force as usual. Forced to make it stop I sighed wondering what Bernard would do next. Offer some exotic Cosmic delight....?

"What do you see?" he said.

"The pyramid. What else?"

"Is that all?

"What am I supposed to see?" I demanded with a slight tone of impatience.

"The plan. Don't you see the plan?" Bernard asked softly and totally patient.

I sensed he really want to scream at me.

"What sort of a plan? Are you suggesting I make a drawing of the Great Pyramid with its insides — the King and Queen Chambers, the passageways...?"

Bernard interrupted. "Just make a simple plan." The sound was now tinged with growing impatience, probably a desire to call me stupid.

"Make a simple plan of the pyramid."

"You're kidding!"

"We never kid. Make a plan," he insisted. "No rulers. Freehand."

Cautiously I did so. Using a pointed black marker on a sheet of ordinary typing paper, I drew a rough square four by four inches.

"How is that?"

"Connect the four corners."

When I had finished it looked like a diagram, a layout of the Great Pyramid. A square crossed by the four edges.

"Now position your pendulum directly above it."

Skeptical, I held the instrument above the drawing. The reaction was immediate: a vigorous swing counter-clockwise!

Totally unbelievable! Challenged, I drew another square and this time inserted a vertical cross instead of the diagonal cross. It brought no response! The pendulum swung limply clockwise.

Curious and given to experimentation I created another square and this time only one line linked two corners. Again, no response. The moment I inserted the missing line making a complete diagonal cross, the pendulum started swinging counter-clockwise.

The conclusion: the diagram has to be in a square with a complete diagonal cross for the process to work.

Another diagram was drawn, this time with the cross strokes failing to meet, in other words the apex, the center cross was missing. The pendulum swung limply clockwise. This means that the square with the completed cross has to be one for pyramid power to flow.

St. Andrew's Cross on the flag of Scotland came to mind. It is a diagonal cross set in a rectangular box. No response! The conclusion is the process only works if the diagonal cross is complete and set in a square. A cross does not work without a square.

It is evident that even without a physical structure of metal, stone, wood and crystal one really does not need a massive great pyramid. Instead a simple plan showing the layout of an X in a roughly drawn square will generate this strange energy — which for now, we'll call Pyramid Power.

One of the circle members suggested the layout is "Cosmic Geometry."

Bernard had his own idea and whispered: "Cosmic Principle. Once you harness the energy of the Principle you can fly anywhere. Think about it."

# THE MISSING CAPSTONE

The capstone, the apex of the Great Pyramid of Giza is missing. In archaeological parlance the word is pyramidion. Any worthy pyramid, particularly the world's greatest and most unique is supposed to have a point, a capstone. But the fact is the Great Pyramid is minus and as we have seen, the plan simply does not work without the center cross, the apex.

At the top of this historic wonder is a flat deck. The Great Pyramid of Giza Research Association points out that the top is flat, in fact visitors can walk around the deck 30 feet in any direction. So why does the monument still insist on showing counter-clockwise energy? The Principle is not complete. Far from it.

The Association raises the obvious question, was the Great Pyramid always without a capstone or was it stolen or possibly destroyed?

Like everything else concerning the Great Pyramid, if the capstone existed it would have been huge and weighed a tremendous amount. As we have seen in experiments a pyramid without a capstone not only loses energy, it fails to work in accordance with the Cosmic Principle.

If you are curious and wish to see a picture of a pyramid with a capstone suspended above it, check the back of a United States dollar bill. The capstone possessing an all-seeing eye is seen detached and floating. Known as the Eye of Providence it appears on many seals, flags, charters and buildings throughout the world. It usually means the "seeing eye" of God but could hark back to the Sumerian clay tablets which referred to god normally flying in the sky or looking down from the sky. This occurs in various instances in the Old Testament which followed the Sumerians by at least a thousand years.

But even without a capstone the Great Pyramid is still attracting and processing energy. A pendulum will swing counter-clockwise over the Google Earth space photo. This created a puzzle, a question. Why? Where was Bernard when one needed him?

Many tourists have endured the difficult climb to the top. One was the esteemed British inventor Sir William Siemens (1823-1883) who founded the still-famous Siemens Engineering business now a global powerhouse.

An Arab guide suggested that if Sir William would raise his hand with fingers outspread, he would hear an acute ringing noise. Raising an index finger, the inventor immediately felt a distinct prickling sensation. Then when he attempted to drink from a bottle of wine he had brought along he received an electric shock. Being an inventor who specialized in electronics, Sir William then moistened a newspaper and wrapped it round a wine bottle and converted it into a Leaden jar — an early form of capacitor. When he held it above his head, it became charged with electricity and immediately, sparks flew from the bottle.

UNHOLY! This terrified Sir William's guides and one of them assumed Siemens was up to some witchcraft so he made a wild attempt to seize the inventor's companion. Promptly, Sir William pointed the bottle towards the Arab and gave him such a shock, it knocked the unfortunate man flat and unconscious on the pyramid deck. When the Arab guide recovered he promptly disappeared, flapping his arms wildly and shouting loudly as he raced down the side of the Great Pyramid.

As the Research Association asks on their website: "What kind of natural phenomena on top of the Great Pyramid could produce such an electrostatic effect?"

One point is very apparent that even without the capstone, the Great Pyramid still generates some form of energy. One wonders what would happen if the missing capstone were found and re-instituted. Probably powerful and enlightening stuff.

Now, is this why many pyramids were built in the world with flat tops or in many cases pyramids were decapitated — simply to neutralize, create a state of dysfunction or plain and simple — switch them off?

The Mayan pyramids of Mexico which were designed with flat tops instead of pointed apexes fail to possess the full Cosmic Principle and this is quickly reflected if a dowser uses a pendulum. It swings clockwise in all cases, which leaves the pondering investigative mind to wonder.

There is one Mexican pyramid with a strange anomaly. The Pyramid of the Sun is the largest building in Teotihuacán and the largest pyramid in Mesoamerica. The name originated with the Aztecs who arrived in the city of Teotihuacán centuries after it was abandoned. Like the Great Pyramid at Giza, the Pyramid of the Sun does not have an apex or pyramidion, but it does have a small platform. At Google Earth if one holds a pendulum over the pyramid it does swing counter-clockwise but sluggishly, even reluctantly.

There are three vast clusters of pyramids in the Nubian Valley of Sudan. These were built by the rulers of the ancient Kushite kingdoms allegedly some 800 years after the pyramids of Ancient Egypt were constructed. Archaeologists surmise that they were copies of the pyramids of Ancient Egypt but on a much lesser scale. One suggestion is the builders must have been frantic to appease the gods or someone in the sky. Approximately 255 smaller pyramids were built over several hundred years

In ancient times all of the pyramid tombs of Nubia were plundered and in recent history the pyramids were further damaged in the 1830s by Egyptian Army deserter, Italian explorer and treasure hunter Giuseppe Ferlini. He blew the tops off at least 40 of the pyramids in the quest for treasure. This mass decapitation blocked any of the pyramids from connecting cosmically.

It raises the question, was Ferlini aware of the Cosmic connection of the pyramids? It is highly doubtful because he was a pure mercenary. He actually found treasure in pyramid N6 at Wad ban Naqa, in the form of dozens of gold and silver jewelry pieces. Upon his return to Europe he catalogued the pieces which were sold and ended up in the State Museum of Egyptian Art at Munich and the Egyptian Museum at Berlin where they remain to this day.

Some of the Nubian pyramids have been rebuilt, but others still stand desecrated, monuments to one man's greed. They can be seen at the Meroe Necropolis north of Khartoum close to the River Nile. The restored pyramids? When tested with a pendulum they function counterclockwise.

Coordinates are 16°56'19.87" N 33°44'55.96" E.

# THE MYSTERIOUS MISSING APEX:

In spite of not having an apex, the Great Pyramid at Giza still functions as if complete. Why? Suddenly the Pyramid's energy took on a new and startling phase.

Throughout history men, women and probably some children have gone to great lengths to explore the Great Pyramid and seek signs of its origin and mystical content. These have been the finest brains in the world and many travelers, adventurers, archaeologists, authors, historians and students have photographed, videotaped, measured, protracted, estimated and theorized over the creature that stands grandly on the Giza Plateau.

Did anyone explore it from a metaphysical point of view? Well, it is highly likely thousands tried something more than just a meditation or prayer session there.

When I started this book I had absolutely no idea that I would be writing these chapters. The original idea was to write a dowser's journey in Northern New York and include parts of Pennsylvania and New Jersey.

So here we are trying to figure out why the Great Pyramid in far off Egypt responds to a pendulum with an insistent counter-clockwise revolution when it is devoid of an apex, a point. Theoretically, it should not work.

As I accosted my newly found friend, Bernard, I did not know that what Betty Lou and I would find would open up a new door in dowsing, healing and cosmic energy and that we were far from finished with the Great Pyramid.

Bernard, a spirit of few words, put it bluntly. "Check the Areas of Influence."

This was not what I wanted to hear. "Bernard, can you help? What was the substance of the missing apex — gold, copper, stone or what?"

My question was ignored because he came up with something entirely different and something I had not even considered.

"Area of Influence. Why don't you measure the area of influence of pyramid energy?"

"Is it important?"

"Do it. Start with the amethyst pyramid on your desk. Place your ruler at the base of the monument then ask your pendulum to indicate the point where the counter-clockwise energy stops and the pendulum commences to move clockwise."

Skeptically, I positioned the one-and-a-half inches tall amethyst pyramid on a part of the open desk top and placed the end of a 12 inch ruler against the base.

Gradually, I moved the swinging pendulum laterally away from the pyramid and along the ruler. It stopped the counter-clockwise rotation at the ten inches mark and started going clockwise.

Fascinated, I held the pendulum on the far side of the little pyramid — same thing.

Dowsers can also perform the reverse. Stand away and gradually approach the pyramid saying: "Show me when the pendulum reaches the outer limits of the Area of Influence of this pyramid." Then measure the point of change. You may be pleasantly surprised.

Curious, the next experiment was with my two-and-a-half inch silver metal pyramid where I expected similar results. The lesson here is not to expect. The pendulum spun counter-clockwise for a distance of 29 inches.

Next, a five-and-a-half inch soapstone pyramid was tested for its area of influence. The pendulum went beyond my 36 inch rule and started going clockwise at approximately four feet.

Bernard for some obscure reason was still working on the Area of Influence and requested a return to Google Earth and the Great Pyramid at Giza.

"Adjust the picture to show the surrounding streets and buildings," urged Bernard. "Now seek the edges of the Area of Influence."

East of the Great Pyramid the pendulum showed the edge was 1.21 km or 0.76 of a mile — Al Mansourey Road, one of the main arteries.

"Your senses may be blocked by a limitation," Bernard commented easily. "It happens. Take a deep breath and relax. Then perform the test again."

My marker started moving east across the Cairo landscape. The pendulum swung counterclockwise for the longest time. Suddenly it stopped and swung clockwise.

"Two-point-five miles or four kilometers!"

"That is not bad for — how did you say? — a crippled pyramid," said Bernard in a soft sarcastic tone.

"Should it be more?"

"Experiment with the Pyramid of Khafre. It possesses a complete edifice."

The pendulum showed Khafre's area of influence was almost twice that of the capless Great Pyramid. The Pharaonic Village and the River Nile are 5.2 miles from the pyramids and the pendulum showed the Area of Influence at four miles.

This was fascinating. "Are you suggesting that if a dowser with a pendulum stands anywhere within a four mile radius of the Khafre Pyramid it will swing only counter-clockwise?"

A soft sigh slipped through the etheric. "If the operator of the pendulum focuses or thinks of the two great monuments, yes. Remember, you are measuring the areas of influence of a certain object."

It was time to ponder and I was trying not to be argumentative.

A complete pyramid built according to the Cosmic Principle, that is a diagonal cross set in a square, only works if it is complete. The masses of decapitated pyramids in the Nubian Valley in the Sudan do not reflect any energy, neither do the square topped pyramids of the Mayan civilization in Mexico.

"Bernard," I said slowly, "Why is the Great Pyramid at Giza defying logic that says the Cosmic Principle has to be complete for it to work?

One could feel grins of sheer amusement occurring on the Other Side.

"Phantom energy." Two words, plain and simple. That was the trouble with Bernard, for a split second the ball was in his court, a moment later is was hurtling back.

"Phantom energy!" I thought. "What's on his mind?"

The subject comes up every time a dowser is asked to search for a missing object, normally a person or more often when a child is lost. It happens. A dowser is called in perhaps days or even a week after a person has disappeared. Meanwhile many people, police, rescue squads, relatives, friends, and teams of volunteers have been scouring the area where they think the person went missing and creating in their own minds scenarios for where the missing person might be.

Each dedicated searcher, probably unaware of the powers of the human mind, creates an energy image so that when the dowser arrives, there is a virtual forest of images — phantom energies — surrounding the search area.

The dowser must then resort to Remanence, a technique developed by the late British dowser Dennis Wheatley which asks the pendulum to show the last actual trail of the missing person. This important technique avoids that forest or jungle of phantom energies.

"Bernard, how does this apply to the Great Pyramid?"

"How many people visit the monument every year?"

"Fourteen million — in normal times."

"How many of them actually see or think of the Great Pyramid as a complete monument?"

"Who knows? Perhaps one per cent," I suggested.

"That's 140,000," said Bernard. "My mathematics indicate that is a substantial number of mindsets generating phantom capstones. If you use Remanence, you'll find the Great Pyramid does not work at all because it is incomplete. However, many people see it as complete and phantom energy makes it so."

"Heavens! I always thought of it as complete," I said.

"Ha! Ha! There you are! You even tricked yourself."

"But wait! That British fellow, Sir William Siemens....," I argued. "Where did he get all that energy to zap the Arab?"

"The Great Pyramid is still very much alive," explained Bernard easily. "It just is not as powerful as the second pyramid Khafre."

"That is your theory why the Great Pyramid at Giza is still alive and creating a large Area of Influence?"

"Do you have a better one?"

# ENERGY AT GIZA – MORE THAN JUST LEYS

It is little wonder that so many great people –warriors, philosophers, states people, generals, pharaohs and even gods from other worlds have been drawn to the Giza Plateau. It is a ley hotspot, similar to Glastonbury and Stonehenge in England, Sedona in Arizona and Mount Ararat in Turkey. But while ley lines have their own attraction, there are other energies contributing in abundance to the focal point at the Great Pyramid.

These are known as geospirals and they are produced by water, usually the result of a phenomenon known as a "blind spring" or a "water dome."

Deep within the Earth there are huge reservoirs of liquids such as oil, natural gas and of course, water. When a reservoir is under pressure, the water is forced upwards through geological faults and appears in the forms of springs. If the water encounters a blockage, an impenetrable rock strata, it becomes "blind" or "domes." Under sustained pressure it seeks ways out through every available rock fissure and results in underground streams and water veins. It is then an energy phenomenon known as geospirals occur.

There are several water domes within the Giza Plateau and archae-ologists have encountered evidence in the form of leakages and springs. For instance when the nearby Tomb of Osiris was excavated in 1944 by Dr Selim Hassan he noted: *"In the eastern side of this hall is yet another shaft about 10.00 m. deep, but unfortunately it is flooded. Through the clear water we can see that it ends in a colonnaded hall, also having side-chambers containing sarcophagi. We tried in vain to pump out the water, but it seems that a spring must have broken through the rock, for continual daily pumping over a period of four years was unable to reduce the water-level. I may add that I had this water analyzed and finding it pure utilized it for drinking purposes." (Hassan 1944: 193)*

Other reports noted similar spring occurrences in deep shafts of the pyramids and tombs. Crews used it for drinking water and some even went swimming in the underground pools.

Geospiral energies are very Yin.

Yin and Yang is a basic concept in traditional Chinese Medicine. It is said to originate 5,000 to 8,000 years ago and is now studied for its pragmatic yet esoteric wisdom. All phenomena are said to be reduced to Yin and Yang. A balanced person is said to be comfortably living Yin and Yang.

Water is Yin. Therefore Yin energy is very relaxing, promotes healing and openly attracts. Pleasant dreams are Yin. It also inspires. Yin is also feminine. Geospirals are Yin.

Dowsing the Great Pyramid reveals at least 18 geospirals working in the sand and limestone immediately underneath and flanking the base. There are two 49-ring geospirals, one to the right side of the north face and the other at the side of the south face. All the others counted showed seven and 14 rings. Together with other blind springs and geospirals, plus leys coming and going, all contribute to the powerful energy force prevailing at these ancient monuments on the Giza Plateau. It is little wonder the place besides being an historic monument and a working vortex attracts more than 14 million visitors a year and many, perhaps unwittingly create the Great Pyramid at Giza with a finished apex.

# MEASURING THE PRINCIPLE IN SPACE

The pyramid, a symbol of ancient times with a message for the future. For generations the inquisitive minds of humanity have attempted to fathom out, rationalize, theorize and speculate on the existence of these great monuments. Lacking imagination they clumsily called them tombs.

Nevertheless millions of people the world over are attracted to the pyramids of Egypt every year. They read or listen to how the ancient slave workers toiled and sweated for years to build the monuments. It is a logical basic human thought pattern. No one really wants to believe there were advanced beings from "somewhere out there" in the Universe who came and colonized Earth and in doing so built key points, such as the Great Pyramid at Giza. As an archaeologist so aptly pointed out all other pyramids are "inferior imitations."

It became evident that the plan of the pyramid concept possesses a healing Yin energy which comes under the title Cosmic Principle. It radiates an energy the field of which can be felt by sensitive humans but also it can be measured through the use of a human holding a pendulum.

If one makes an eight by eight inch drawing of the plan of a pyramid which Spirit calls the Cosmic Principal, this too produces a large Area of Influence. An experimenter can draw a pyramid plan of any dimension. The smaller it is, the smaller the Area of Influence. The larger the drawing, the larger the Area of Influence. There must be a formula, but we have not to this point discovered it. Perhaps some academically oriented dowsers can work on this.

So far it is apparent the bigger the pyramid or indeed the drawn diagram which Bernard calls the Cosmic Principle, the more volume and area the energy covers. The only measuring tools we have are the pendulum and the human consciousness. Using these we discover that the Principle's energy does not just flow as a simple column above and below the format, but radiates a wide lateral influence.

But what of vertical influence. Is that similar to the reaches of the influence laterally? Apart from standing on an eleven foot tall ladder and checking a mini-pyramid we have no further confirmation.

Somewhere in our research someone came up with the suggestions that a vertical Area of Influence may not be limited. It was supposed the pyramid acted as a conduit and allowed energy to flow one way or the other, at least that was the idea at first. So it was back to Google Earth with a pendulum and pointer looking down on the Great Pyramid.

"We are seeking the upper limits of energy of the Great Pyramid," I said to the pendulum and my higher consciousness. This is one of the very useful attributes manifested by Google Earth. It displays the elevation from which you are viewing.

A pendulum at 10,625 feet above the Great Pyramid showed a strong response. Enthused we took the viewpoint up to 23,000 feet. The pendulum played dead. Not a hint. So there was an upper limit. We reduced the viewpoint down to 16,883 feet. Still no response. 12,000 — no response. We returned to 10,625 feet. A full response.

Somewhere between 10,625 and 12,000 feet, just over two miles the Area of Influence of the Great Pyramid ceases.

"Test the second pyramid at Giza — Khafre. It is complete," Bernard suggested mildly.

A few minutes later we were finished measuring. "The pendulum registers energy but feebly at 23,000 feet but nothing at all at 30,920," I said. "That's over four miles. Double the Great Pyramid."

"The cornerstone, the apex makes a great difference," said Bernard with a nod. "Your so-called phantom energies don't really help."

"Oh, it shows the Great Pyramid, the grand-father of them all, still has a power in spite of being decapitated," I said, then added: "That's enough vertical influence for a visiting alien space traveler to sit with a pendulum and know he or she is on target."

Bernard was quiet for some seconds, then he said: "If space travelers were that advanced thousands of years ago, they probably had a robot crew member who was Cosmic Principle sensitive."

"There will always be human dowsers," I protested.

"With the way your people are advancing with artificial intelligence, the coming of robot dowsers is simply a matter of time."

"With a Higher Consciousness? Do you think…" I started to say.

The only question remaining is the date," said Bernard.

But there was little time for us to think because he was about to reveal another development.

# PYRAMID POWER ON PAPER

It happened one dark wintry evening and I was alone in my study wondering about the Great Pyramid and Bernard's revelation of vertical force. My hand reached for that original four inch drawing I had made some moons before. I could still hear his sharp cultured voice. "The plan! Draw the plan of the pyramid. No rulers! Freehand!"

The simplicity was powerful, difficult to comprehend. "Why? Why? Why? Like all pyramid stuff, an answer generates more questions. I gazed at the piece of paper containing the roughly drawn plan.

For centuries many good people have looked in awe at the Great Pyramid and wondered, theorized, measured and supposed why it was there. Now I was staring at a roughly drawn plan — a simple black inked square with a diagonal cross inside.

A gentle breeze drafted through on my right side. It was Bernard with his down to Earth questioning. "What do you see now, Mr. Egby?"

"A square with a diagonal cross," I said refusing to acknowledge he was now calling me mister instead of plain Egby.

"Look again!

"Every angle in the diagram is either 45 or 90 degrees," I said.

"Four and five are nine and ninety is nine anyway," he added.

"It's the Cosmic Nine," I put in. "All the folks who measured the insides and outsides concluded that all measurements of the Great Pyramid reduce to the Cosmic Nine."

"Absolutely! Now draw the figure nine."

Grabbing the black marker I scribbled a nine and held a pendulum over it. Counter-clockwise!

"Now draw an eight." Clockwise!

"A seven...a six...a five..." He rattled them off as I drew and the pendulum swirled clockwise.

"Now place a one in front of the eight to make it 18."

"Counter-clockwise!

"Bernard, so any number that adds or reduces to nine will bring about a counter-clockwise reaction," I said.

My Spirit friend was not finished.

"Hold your finger on the nine and at the same time hold the pendulum over it."

It swung counter-clockwise.

"Slowly move up and away."

The pendulum kept swinging until it was about two inches away. Still it was two inches.

"Area of Influence," noted Bernard. "Now do the same thing over your sketch."

The pendulum swung counter-clockwise over the drawing and continued to do so as it was pulled away. With mixed feelings of skepticism and wonderment I watched the swinging pendulum. It finally stopped about 30 inches from the drawing and commenced a clockwise rotation..

"Area of influence," said Bernard with a brief chuckle

"This changes things a lot. Do you mean to tell me a roughly drawn plan of a pyramid on a piece of paper can generate Yin energy," I asked, trying not to sound skeptical.

"Did you not do it?"

"Sure! So moving further along this crazy path of oddball logic," I put the question: "So why do we have pyramids if all we need is a Cosmic Plan?"

"Principle!" said the voice. "It's a Principle."

"Fine! It sounds snotty. A Cosmic Principal," I muttered. "Has anybody bothered to use your Principle on a large scale?"

"You might try the Kazakhs, some mystical people who inhabit the northern parts of Central Asia," said the voice slowly. "The Principle is even larger in size than the Great Pyramid."

# THE PRINCIPLE ON THE ASIAN STEPPES

Republic of Kazakhstan set in Central Asia is the world's largest landlocked country by land area and the ninth largest country in the world. It has vast mineral resources along with oil and gas. It borders Russia, China, Kyrgyzstan, Uzbekistan, and Turkmenistan and also adjoins a large part of the Caspian Sea. It has every terrain imaginable — flatlands, steppe, taiga, rock canyons, hills, deltas, snow-capped mountains, and deserts. Close to 20 million people, many descendants of the great Mongol tribes, live there. The capital is Astana and the country's news suddenly jolted the world's archaeological fraternity in a challenging way in 2007.

That is when satellite pictures of a remote and barren treeless zone on the northern steppes revealed a community of earthworks including squares, crosses, lines and rings which like the Peruvian Nazca Lines can only be seen from the air — or really in space. Estimates consider the site to be at least 8,000 years old.

While using Google Earth what caught the eye of Kazakh economist and dedicated archaeological explorer Dmitriy Dey were the various mounds, earthworks, trenches all designed in five basic shapes, miles from anywhere.

One of the shapes formed a distinct square with the corners linked together to form a diagonal cross. The Cosmic Principle!

Archaeologists call it the Ushtogaysky Square.

The size of this square is about eight hectares or 20 acres which makes it infinitely larger than the Great Pyramid's base area of 13 acres. The square consists of 101 mounds. The 101st is located in the center. On each side are 15 barrows and 10 barrows in each half-diagonal.

The discovery was detailed in 2014 at an archaeological conference in Istanbul because it was new and previously unstudied. Some traditional archaeologists suggested "fake" and "hoax" but Dr. Ronald LaPorte, a University of Pittsburgh scholar with the help of an American health coordinator in Kazakhstan tracked down Mr. Dey who quickly provided images and documents to convince the conference of its authenticity.

The site is in danger of highway developers and local authorities are being urged to seek protection from the United Nations Educational, Scientific and Cultural Organization . One ancient figure known as the Koga Cross was damaged if not destroyed by road builders.

One major point that appears to have been settled by archaeologists, the site was not a cenotaph or any place for preserving the dead.

The Ushtogaysky Square is available for all to see on Google Earth. Simply put the name into the program's Search Box. Once you have the picture on your computer or laptop, take a pendulum and see how it swings. It is a power house: counter-clockwise!

This of course raises some questions

Did the ancient builders of the site and the square in particular know and understand what they were doing? Had they heard of the Great Pyramid in Egypt and were attempting to build one themselves by laying out the groundwork? Or did they know of the Cosmic Yin energy manifested by the design — the Cosmic Principle? If so, who or what was their source of information? Why was it created in the middle of the barren Asian Steppes? Does the design have an Area of Influence?

The answer to the last question is a definite affirmative. The Area of Influence of the Ushtogaysky Square is substantial — a task for future dowsers or open minded archaeologists with pendulums. For physical and digital dowsers the coordinates are: 50°49′58.96" N and 65°19′34.44" E.

# EXPLORING THE COSMIC PRINCIPLE

As we have seen a 2.5 inch metal pyramid radiates an energy field spanning approximately 10 inches. A 5 inch sandstone pyramid radiates a field of about 24 inches. As dowsed earlier, the Areas of Influence of the two major pyramids at Giza extend over several miles. It would be interesting to discover the formula — if such a thing exists. One noticeable factor: Areas of Influence appear to change fractionally, perhaps according to the weather, lunar phases or something else.

Right now, let us pursue the Cosmic Principle and transfer the diagram of a square inset with a diagonal cross to paper.

For a test we drew an eight inch square with a diagonal cross on a regular sheet of paper. Standing by itself its Area of Influence was eleven feet or four paces. The author's pace is 33 inches.

For the collective test nine copies were made and placed in a three by three alignment on a table close to open doors with the yard and forest beyond.

My surmising thought was that if one pyramid plan produces four paces, nine should produce an energy force measurable by a pendulum swinging counterclockwise for 36 paces.

In the test the pendulum swung counter-clockwise for 43 paces up to the line of the first trees. This would be 1,419 inches or 118.25 feet. The collective difference? Eight paces or 22 feet.

Remember, this collective Area of Influence is being measured only by radius. The total area covered is just over one acre or 43,560 square feet.

The Area of Influence of one eight inch square pyramid plan is 379.94 *square feet.*

In other words, the more pyramids you draw (or build), the greater the Area of Influence. As mentioned before, in their heyday the Nubian pyramids totaling several hundred would have projected a magnificent force, perhaps too much. For one reason or another many were decapitated and consequently lost much of their powers. Again, did someone know of the Cosmic Principle and wanted the monuments crippled? Who knows? It is good to hear that some have been rebuilt.

Did the Nubians build a multiplicity of pyramids because they knew of the force that exists in the Cosmic Principle? I was mulling this over when Bernard finally dropped in.

"Robert, when you draw or copy a Principle, it becomes a conductor. No matter where you place it, it will always radiate a column of energy. Each one operates in its own space and time. "

"But it compounds."

"That's true," he said. "If you have nine fountains you will have nine times as much water."

"So what's the true purpose of this Cosmic Energy?"

"Ha! That's for you to find out," said the voice with a chuckle. "If you can."

"That's hard. For some time I imagined you were here to assist," I muttered.

"Oh, foolish expectations," chided Bernard easily sounding a little Dickensian. "All's well, so why don't you talk about the healing powers of the Principle." It was more of a statement than a question.

## USING THE PRINCIPLE FOR HEALING

The reader will recall that in our early explorations it was found that model pyramids can reduce discomforts such as arthritis and muscle aches but the problem is such models are difficult to handle. Even though one student who suffered problems in her hand exclaimed as she held a mini-pyramid: "I can feel some relief in my joint." Several others voiced remarks such as "I feel better, more energized just holding it. Isn't that strange?"

"Heavens above!" exclaimed Bernard. "They do not have to hold a physical pyramid. Tell them to draw the Principle and sit in its Area of Influence."

A piece of paper with something drawn on it can heal? It sounds plain crazy to many people. The idea that one take a drawing of the Cosmic Principle and sit in its Area of Influence sounded strange and impractical to some people. Some initially thought the idea of a drawn Principle taped over a part of the human body suffering pain and stress sounded plain dumb, if not stupid. However, unbeknown to myself, destiny was to play a role in this.

While working in the yard in New Jersey my enthusiastic gardening partner Betty Lou, just 81 at the time, picked up a 40 lb bag of top soil the wrong way. Result: a couple of compressed fractures in her spinal column. After an Emergency visit to the local hospital, she was committed to spending a lot of days on the couch. Taking a dislike to the effects of prescribed medicine she asked if pyramid energy would help heal.

I have long been a follower of the decrees of the Biblical Prophet Job. The Bible says: "You will also decree a thing, and it will be established for you; And light will shine on your ways."

In dowsing workshops when inclement weather insists on participants staying and working indoors, we have often decreed energy zones such as geopathic lines for search and demonstration purposes. This is a common practice taught many years ago by veteran Canadian dowser Tom Passey.

Tom called them "phantoms" and to all intents and purposes they existed. The important thing to remember when you have created phantoms is clean up afterwards: Decree phantom energies neutralized, gone.

Rejecting pain killers Betty Lou needed some healing and relief, so with her permission I decreed a large phantom pyramid suspended over her body as she lay on the couch with her two Chihuahua companions. Naturally, I tested its existence with a pendulum and received confirmation by a vigorous counter-clockwise swing.

Next day Betty Lou reported that while she felt much better, she had experienced some "strange" dreams and the dogs were now so lazy, they acted as if they had been drugged. The phantom pyramid was too much and so it was eliminated.

In its place I drew the plan of the Cosmic Principle measuring about four by four inches on a small piece of paper. Betty Lou tucked this into her clothes over the affected pain area. The diagram stayed for several days and she reported it helped her "feel much better," but complained it kept on moving or falling off, even when taped.

Eventually we found a blue skin marker and drew a Cosmic Principle plan, about four by four inches covering the point of the discomfort. We did this almost daily until she felt well enough to do without. Each day we used a pendulum to check its validity and effectiveness.

Once while checking on this technique Bernard came through and said it was not only reducing the discomfort of a painful condition but its area of influence was keeping Betty Lou relaxed. Incidentally, she informed her doctor on all of this and he nodded: "Good idea. Keep it up."

# PRINCIPLE HEALING: HOW TO DO IT

This is a delicate chapter so I will make it barebones and simple. Once you are an accomplished dowser and sensitive to energies, you may wish to try and experience this next exercise for yourself.

Find a comfortable space such as a bed, sofa, recliner or even a mat on the floor where you will eventually lie down and relax and do whatever you wish to do. Perhaps your goal is to experience lucid dreams, recuperate from a sickness or generally reboot your creative energies for writing a book, painting a picture or taking photographs, or just to hang out in total peace.

Before conducting this exercise make sure you have not been drinking alcohol and you feel clean in both body and mind.

Now sit on a regular chair and relax for a few moments by concentrating on your body breathing. As you focus, your breathing will slow down and get you into the alpha meditation stage.

Then when you feel ready look at the comfortable place in front of you and say in a firm authoritative voice: *"In the name of the Cosmic Forces* (you can use Holy Spirit, God, Infinite Intelligence, the Creator or whoever you pray to) *I decree that a pyramid six feet by six feet and three feet tall, true to the Cosmic Principle be created and exist in front of me. It is for my health and learning. I ask this in Your Name. Amen and So Be It."*

The wording does not have to be identical to the above, but the intent is critically important. If you wish to enhance the decree, see or imagine that pyramid in front of you. If you are prone to clairvoyance or psychometry you will likely see a pyramid.

When you are ready, take a pendulum and see which way it swings. If you have executed the command properly it will swing counter-clockwise and build up a forceful response. It is then you can leave your chair and lie down inside your pyramid and meditate, dream, and bathe in the healing, energies and all those things. If you have a medical condition tell your professional health practitioner about your pyramid.

The above exercise is very useful if you are recuperating after an operation or medical treatments that might be arduous. An experienced dowser can also decree a pyramid for others in need. If you do always monitor the condition and remove if necessary.

When you feel accomplished, the decreed pyramid can be very useful as a metaphysical development center for classes. One thing you cannot teach under the Cosmic Principle is dowsing with a pendulum. It may not be obvious but in order to perform dowsing exercises on other things outside the pyramid it is difficult, if not impossible simply because of the pyramid's Yin energy. It is like trying to teach someone how to swim when they are sitting at the bottom of a river.

One more thing. Draw an eight by eight inch square on a sheet of paper, include a diagonal cross, then make sure it is intact by holding a pendulum over it. It will swing counter-clockwise. Then place it in your bedroom and forget it. You may experience some vivid dreams for the first few nights, then deep sleep with interesting dreams coming through.

Test the Area of Influence with a pendulum. If you wish to cover your entire house, make multiple copies of the drawing and staple them together. Place the bundle in a safe place then walk through your house or apartment with a pendulum and check the Area of Influence. You may well be surprised at the coverage.

Do not use this in place of treatment for a recognized condition by a professional medical or health practitioner. Use it as an adjunct to regaining good health.

# THE PRINCIPLE'S POWER ON PLANTS

In parallel research the powers of a casually drawn pyramid plan on a sheet of paper became intriguing in other ways. In our Zen Room which serves as a classroom and workshop, Betty Lou's son, Ken maintained a veritable array of green vegetation including a trio of three Spider plants (Chlorophytum comosum) growing in small clay pots by the window. When we tried our first experiment with the Cosmic Principle the Spider plants were small and still young.

A four inch pyramid diagram was placed under the middle plant. The idea was to see if that plant's growth could be changed by simple paper pyramid energy. It was an early experiment and at this point I had yet to discover the phenomenon known as an Area of Influence. It was a learning experience.

In a month the three plants all showed distinct and healthy growth, in fact they had not only grown upwards, seventeen inches instead of the normal maximum of twelve, the roots had expanded and cracked the sides of the clay pots. Not just one here, another there, but all three on the same day! It was truly stunning. Ken repacked the three in larger clay pots.

If you are going to experiment use a small drawing of perhaps an inch under a selected plant. Or do what we should have done in the first place, discover the Area of Influence and once established move other plants away. Check with a pendulum.

If you are a dowser or have a partner with gardening talents this could be a great area for research. Do not forget to keep a detailed journal and take photographs. Your local gardening club might like to hear of your exploits, including your dowsing notes.

# PLASTIC THE TRADITIONAL ENERGY BLOCKER

Many dowsers are aware that plastic sheets are psychic energy blockers. If you encounter a "runaway psychic" — someone who has abilities but cannot control them — here is a temporary remedy. Place a small patch of plastic over the person's solar plexus and all manifestations will cease. Any grocery shopping bag will do, simply cut a small square six by six inches, bigger if the person is larger, and tape it onto the solar plexus chakra, the point in the body immediately below the belly button. The same if someone is hallucinating. Place a plastic patch over the center of the head, the crown chakra and visions will cease. This is a temporary technique for use until the person gets to a professional therapist for treatment.

Plastic garbage bags will also block geopathic energy for about three months before its blocking powers deteriorate.

Bearing this in mind and armed with a pendulum we placed a mini-pyramid inside a plastic shopping bag and half-expected a complete block. Surprise! The pendulum's swing was so powerful it was as if the plastic did not exist. It swung vigorously counter-clockwise. Apparently the Cosmic Principle overrides where psychic energy fails.

During the next few months various ideas crossed our minds, usually instigated by Bernard who seemed to delight in intruding when I am studying or researching something else.

While the Great Pyramid of Giza may have been a marker for ancient travelers and was built to a simple Cosmic formula — a diagonal cross inside a square? We know it manifests relaxing and healing energies, so what other uses and powers does it possess?

**Unless otherwise stated all photographs are by the author.**

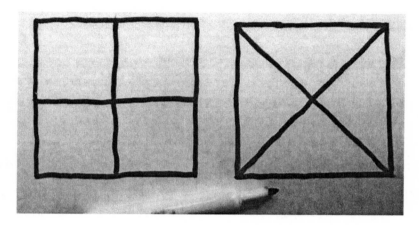

THE ORIGINAL DRAWING of the Cosmic Principle by the author. A cross with a diagonal square. The regular cross in a square was an immediate test of the Spirit's suggestion and it failed. Use a pendulum over the right picture and it immediately goes counter-clockwise. The square is of course the plan of a pyramid.

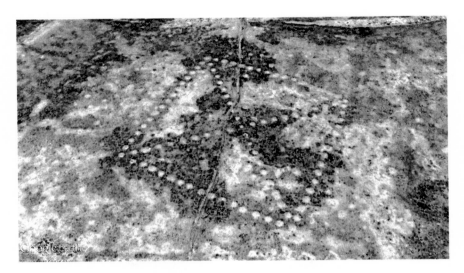

THE PLAN OF A PYRAMID IN DEEPEST ASIA. Discovered in 2014, it covers 20 acres compared to the Great Pyramid at Giza's 13 acres. Named the Ushtogaysky Square, it comprises 101 mounds and can be found in the Republic of Kazakhstan. Yes, it forms a Comic Principle and it generates a counter-clockwise swing of the pendulum. Credit: Google Earth Pro.

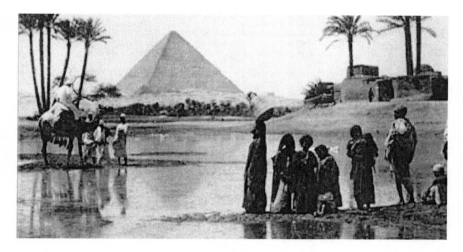

THE GREAT PYRAMID AT GIZA scanned from a 19<sup>th</sup> Century Stereopticon card shows the scene as the author recalls it in the early 1950s — not many tourists. Credit: Public domain but scanned by Infrogmation.

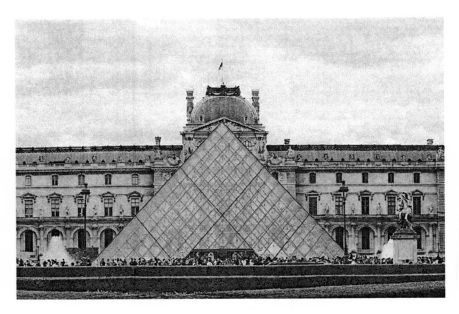

PYRAMID AND LEYS IN PARIS. If you are standing exactly where this photograph was taken, you are standing on one of two three-haired leys that converge on the Pyramid built as an entrance to the famous Louvre. Photo: Alvesgaspar - Own work, CC BY-SA 3.0, commons.wikimedia.org/w/index.php?curid=16126578

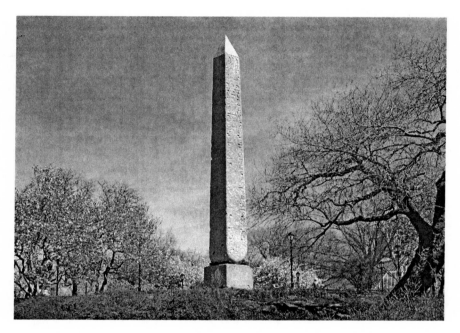

AN EGYPTIAN OBELISK IN CENTRAL PARK. It is 3,500 years old, 69 feet tall, weighs 220 tons and is often called "Cleopatra's Needle" by mistake. Between the Obelisk and the nearby Metropolitan Museum of Art runs the Fifth Avenue ley. Photo: Ken Kishler.

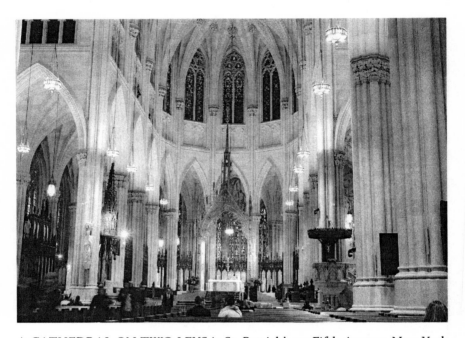

A CATHEDRAL ON TWO LEYS is St. Patrick's on Fifth Avenue, New York City. The two leys cross where the Nave and the Transept meet. This energy accompanied by several geospirals is a great place to relax, pray and do some creative thinking. Photo: Ken Kishler

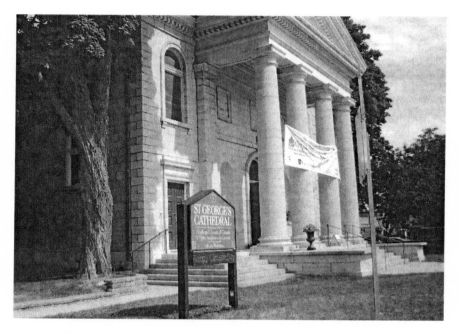

A CANADIAN CATHEDRAL WITH ENERGY. This is St. George's Anglican on King Street East in Kingston, Ontario. It has a leyline that crosses the front doors. We discovered it by accident while tracking a US-Canada ley across the street that passes through the Diocesan Offices and Bookshop. This picture is interesting in that the tree is twisted, a sign of a geopathic zone in spite of being on a ley. Photo: Robert Egby

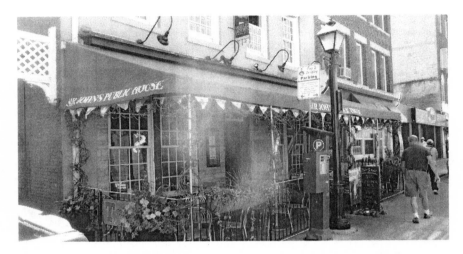

A PLACE FOR HIGH SPIRITS? While dowsing on Kingston's King Street East we followed the ley as it tracked through some buildings, including one that served as an office for Canada's first prime minister, Sit John A. Macdonald. As we walked by I snapped a picture. Now it's known as Sir John's Public House. The photograph is odd, some might say it is a spirit manifesting. Take a peek.

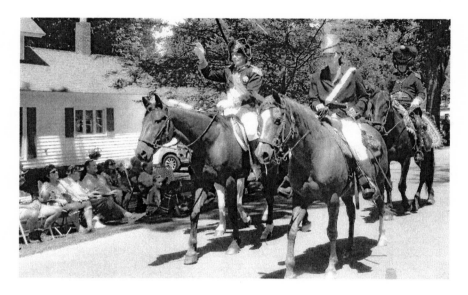

CAPE VINCENT AND THE FRENCH CONNECTION. Back in the early 1800s a group of French exiles gathered in secret to rescue Emperor Napoleon imprisoned by the British on the remote Atlantic island of St, Helena. It never happened, but over almost half a century Cape Vincent has celebrated an annual French Festival in Early July. Napoleon, played by Ron Jacobs rides with an entourage cheered by the crowds. Photo: Robert Egby

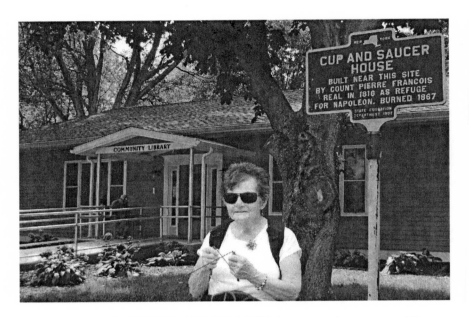

NAPOLEONIC PLOTTERS MET ON A LEY. A spacious house resembling an inverted cup and saucer was built for the Emperor. The house has long gone and today Cape Vincent's Community Library shares part of the property. Betty Lou dowses a ley line on site. Photo: Robert Egby

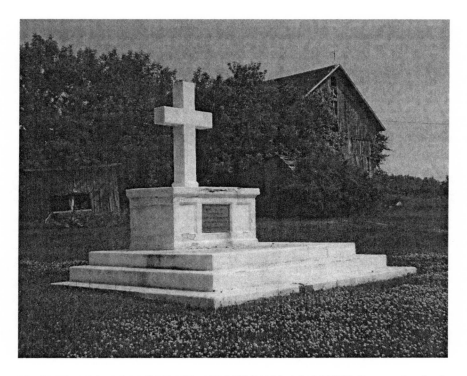

TUCKED AWAY IN UPSTATE NEW YORK IS A VORTEX. Passers by don't often stop at this white memorial altar. The sign reads: French Catholic Church. Built here in 1832 by early settlers. Heroes of Napoleon's Army and French Refugees worshiped here. The church has long gone but the site contains 19 geospirals with an Area of Influence well over half a mile — covering the Veterans resting in the nearby cemetery. Photo: Robert Egby

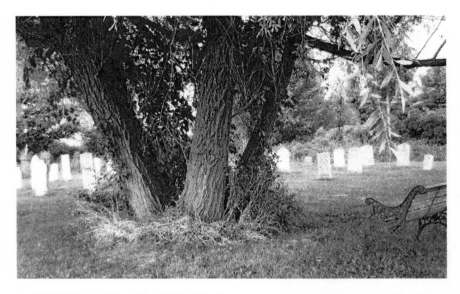

A GEOSPIRAL IN A GRAVEYARD. Dowsers can recognize geospiral locations by observing trees — they flourish like these in the Rosiere French and German Pioneers Cemetery in upstate New York. Photo: Robert Egby

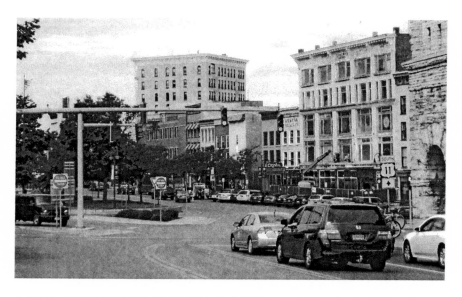

A KEG OF ENERGY IN WATERTOWN NY. For those who know, sitting on the island in the middle of the Square is a joy to behold. It should be because no less than four leys sweep through the place and this makes it an attraction for arts, crafts, writers, photographers and various schools such as music. Such a gathering of leys can sorely test any dowser. Photo Robert Egby

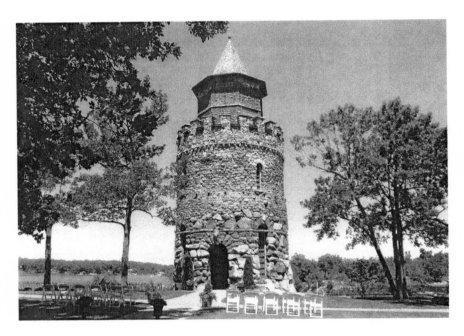

THIS IS THE DOVECOTE AT BOLDT CASTLE which sits in the middle of the St. Lawrence River. It is here couples get married and a great place to launch a wedded life — it is on a ley that starts in Canada, passes through the exact center of the Dovecote, then heads off for Alexandria Bay Hospital and Watertown beyond. Photo Robert Egby

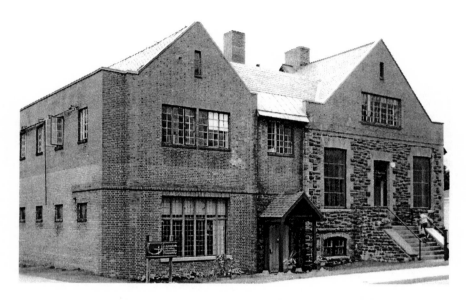

A MAN WITH A MISSION worked in this building in a northern New York mountain town named Saranac Lake during the last part of the 19th century and well into the 20th century. His name Dr. Edward Trudeau and he ran a dedicated village of rest and recuperation for people suffering from Consumption or Tuberculosis. This was his laboratory and a ley line runs through it. In fact it is the longest ley line in North America. Photo Robert Egby

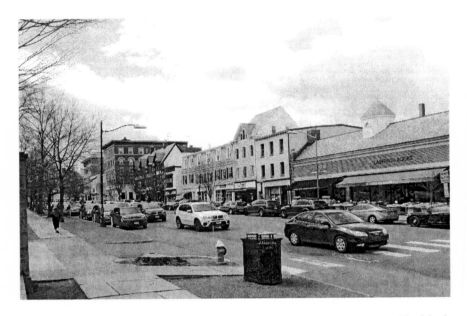

NASSAU STREET IN PRINCETON at a point where two leys cross. The black car on the crosswalk marks the spot. One ley from the Princeton Cemetery crosses into the University (at left) and a ley flowing along Nassau gradually completes the crossing at Palmer Square entrance. Photo: Robert Egby

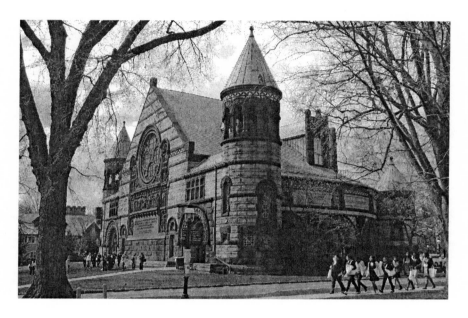

FOUR LEYS CROSS PRINCETON accompanied by numerous geospirals make it a great place for studying and creation. This is one several elegant and impressive buildings in the town. It's the Richardson Auditorium in the Alexander Hall. Photo Robert Egby

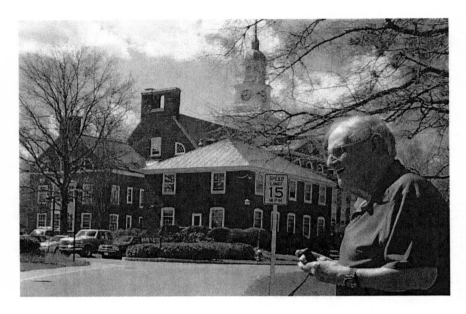

A STATELY HOME FOR ADVANCED MINDS. This is where such great thinkers as Einstein, Oppenheimer, Panofsky and Goldman came and worked. It's the Institute for Advanced Studies. The author stands on the ley as it moves towards the Institute. Photo: Betty Lou Kishler

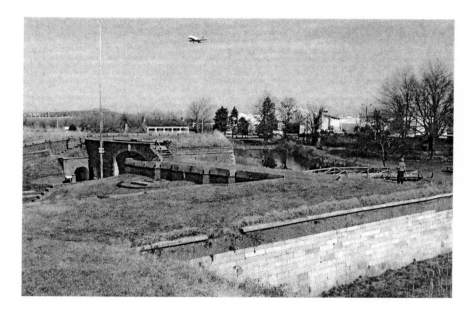

A REMNANT OF THE WAR OF INDEPENDENCE. Fort Mifflin is the only military base in use that is older than the nation itself. On the Delaware river and close to Philadelphia International Airport it played key roles. It is known for its unusual battlements designed by Pierre L'Enfant who laid out Washington, DC. Photo Robert Egby

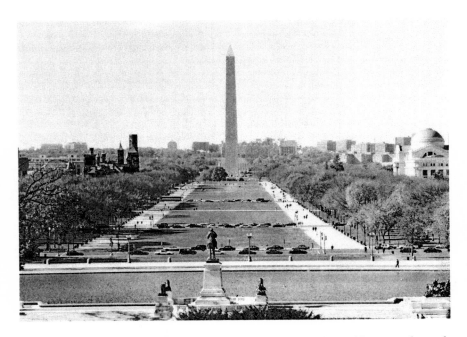

A VIEW FROM THE CAPITOL BUILDING — A triple-haired ley runs through the seat of Government, through the Ulysses S. Grant Memorial along the middle of the National Mall, and on to the Washington Monument and beyond towards Arlington. The monument, although built in the USA conforms to the Cosmic Principle.

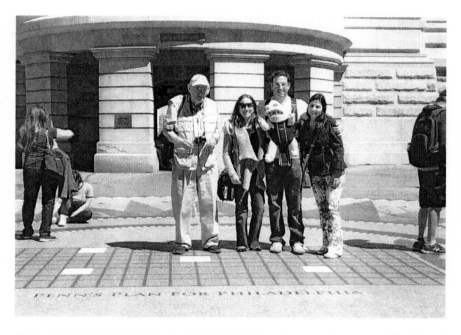

PHILADELPHIA CITY HALL COURTYARD where two leys cross. The Broad
Street ley and the Market Street ley. William Penn's complete alignment. A
visiting Brazilian family joined the author for a photo at the crossing. Observe
others in the photo. A young man stands quietly waiting, two young people, one
seated on the tiles, the other stands. That's the attraction of leys and geospirals.
Photo: Betty Lou Kishler

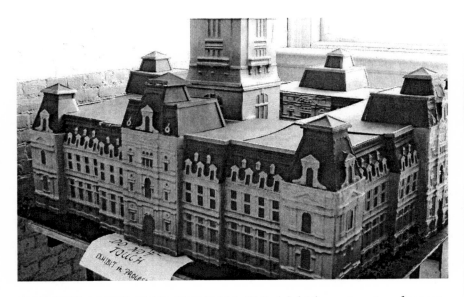

EIGHT PYRAMIDS ATOP CITY HALL. Philadelphia's great center of government building boasts eight Cosmic Principle pyramids on the roof. Difficult to photograph, it is made easy by this model inside the building. Incidentally, even the staircase posts in City Hall have bronze mini-pyramids.

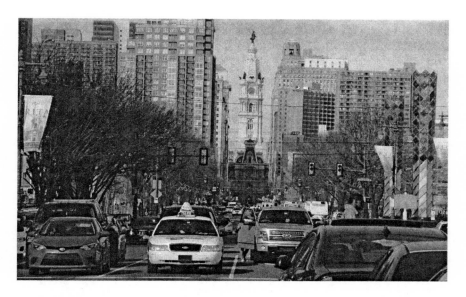

THE BROAD STREET LEY TRAVELS SOUTH in the middle of the street.
William Penn atop City Hall looks on. By the time the ley gets to the Naval
Yard it is on the east side. This position is outside The National Shrine of St.
Rita of Cascia.

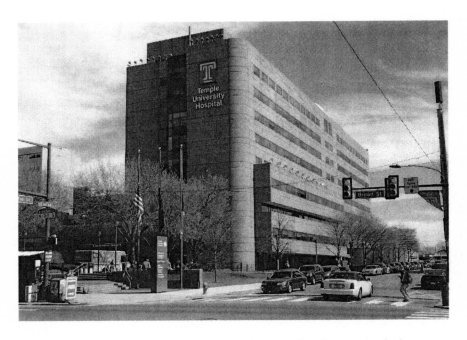

DID RUSSELL CONWELL FEEL THE ENERGY when he acquired a house on Philadelphia's North Broad? The author of "Acres of Diamonds" taught recognition of good things and started Temple University. The site is now home to Temple Hospital.

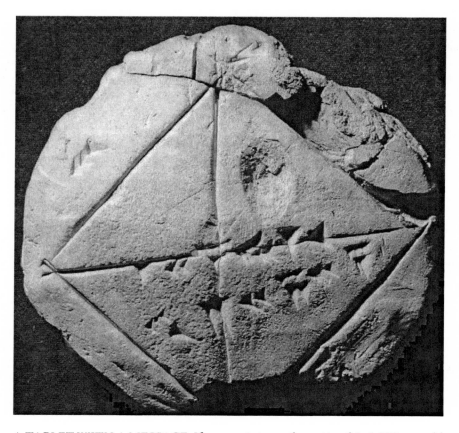

A TABLET WITH A MESSAGE. If you are into mathematics this 6,000 year old Sumerian tablet is a prize. Look further and it contains the Cosmic Principle, a square with a diagonal cross, the plan of a pyramid. Try your pendulum on this picture. Credit: Bill Casselman, photographer/ math.ubc.ca

# BOOK THREE

## SEARCHING FOR THE PRINCIPLE IN THE WEST

Pyramids! The Cosmic Principle! Ley lines and Geospirals. They are all Earth and Cosmic energies. That particular sentence is wrong. For instance it is easy to find people who think the Cosmos and Cosmic are "things out there" in space. The truth is Earth is part of space, the Universe, the Milky Way galaxy. Whether we like it or not, we and Planet Earth are all Cosmic, so enjoy.

In a moment of philosophy Bernard said "Every garden, every backyard, every home, every office, every part of life on your planet is wrapped up and benefitting from Cosmic energies. There is not a blade of grass or the smallest grain of sand that is not Cosmic."

Suddenly we became aware that we needed to find Principle phenomena in the Americas. Initially, it seemed a difficult and indeed a challenging mission. How many pyramids are available in the country? Initially it seemed difficult but when we became "pyramid conscious" they sprang up in countless places.

In Vancouver-Richmond in Canada's British Columbia I was scheduled to do a workshop and wanted to perform a pyramid demonstration. Betty Lou helped search all the gift shops, novelty stores and New Age places in the various centers. One shopkeeper said: "I usually have a couple here. My wife says they're spooky, so I haven't re-ordered." He was amazed when I provided a five minute wrap on pyramid energy. "I'll have to tell her," he said with a grin.

After an all-day search we found a Himalayan salt pyramid in Steveston New Age shop and it worked like a charm. Then in the ensuing weeks we started to notice pyramids in real places.

If when traveling observe buildings — homes and commercial — and you may well find a pyramid shaped roof with four sides and an apex at the top. While in New Jersey for the winter we spotted a pyramid almost every time we were out. Several were on business fronts such as a health spa on Lumberton's Route 38, an automotive center on the Mount Holly-Burlington Road and another on top of an aging shack in Pemberton Township. Several homes have rooftops showing complete pyramids — that is four sloping sides connected at the top in a pointed apex — and one wonders what it must be like living in such places. Does one ever get sick living under a Principle? Are inhabitants unusually healthy? Has a child raised under a pyramid roof gone on to become a celebrity on the highway of life?

Philadelphia has many pyramids. There's a whole cluster of eight good sized ones on the roof at City Hall and inside the historic building on the staircases small brass pyramids cap the posts at the ends of hand rails.

In Northern New York there's an almost free standing pyramid over the entrance to the Salmon Run Mall in Watertown. Unless you know what it means, few people passing by fail to look up or even pause under the roof to enjoy the energy. But nevertheless it is there and if a pendulum is available it always swings counter-clockwise.

Pyramid energy or Cosmic Principle while it is freely available for everyone for some it is not the easiest gift of the Universe to live with or handle. For creative folk it motivates writing, artwork such as painting, sculpture, carving, music and singing, it also provokes lucid dreaming and feelings of well-being. While it is beneficial and creates a wonderful living style for many people, it can be too much of a good thing. It can assist and bolster any tendency that grips your life.

For instance if a person or a family living or working under the Cosmic Principle possesses a tendency towards laziness, negative thinking and living it will actually intensify such behavior until one has to break out of the influence or seek positive change through Yang activities.

The best way to handle a home or an office that is under a Cosmic Principle influence is to be conscious of it, appreciate its existence and go with the flow. It happened with that very unusual and creative architect Michael E. Reynolds who lives in Taos, New Mexico.

A proponent of "radically sustainable living" he is known for the design and construction of the internationally recognized "Earthship" passive solar homes. Construction reuses unconventional building materials from waste sources such as automobile tires. His designs test the limits of building codes.

Fresh out of architecture school at the University in Cincinnati in 1969, Michael Reynolds moved to Taos. During earlier vacations he had spent time in the area and "loved it." He had heard that the mountain of the Pueblo Indians was one of the power spots on the planet. Once in Taos he never wanted to leave. "Something happened to me here. I felt so at home that I think I must have stumbled onto my own energy," he writes in his book *A Coming of Wizards*.

He explains: "What I mean is, I found that particular state of mind which allows the oneness or wholeness of the universe to prevail over human dogma. I believe this state of mind is a key to the limitless energy of the universe."

Enthralled with pyramids he created a large perfectly scaled one on top of his house and positioned his bed right at the King's Chamber. As he lay there, he became acutely conscious that he was sleeping in a "beautiful valley at the base of a sacred power mountain, in a land so akin to my essence of my own being that I felt like it ran in my body, through my veins and out again."

It was in the early 1970s while in the pyramid that he began having "intense experiences, dreams, instances of automatic writing and outright visions." He stresses he was not on any drug, alcohol or other mind altering substance when one afternoon he was lying on his back in the pyramid and he experienced a spiritual visitation by four wizards.

"They clearly and vividly made me aware of a way of seeing and moving that grows in potential through use, with apparently infinite resonance," he says.

Adopting cautious consideration at first, he began to find similarities between their information, eastern mysticism and quantum physics, the ways of the Shaman, the nature of plants and animals and the processes of the planet itself. As he became more focused about the information, "I found myself on a journey to a world that reflects more than just the human condition." His thoughts, realizations and an upward change in consciousness are explained in his fascinating and inspiring book *A Coming of Wizards.*

In 1972 he built his first house from recycled materials. He utilized everyday discarded trash items like aluminum cans, plastic bottles and used tires. In place of conventional and energy-consuming recycling methods he used them as-is. He realized that any container and object, be it a soda bottle or an old tire, could be transformed into a powerful and durable insulation when filled with dirt. He calls this practice Earthship Biotecture and he has dedicated his life to it and authored at least five books on it.

If one heads out of Taos and crosses the great Rio Grande bridge which is 650 feet above the river and heads west a short distance on U.S. Route 64 the traveler will find Michael Reynold's work. It's called Earthship Taos. Incidentally, if you live overseas, you may have one in your country.

## THE ANCIENT GREAT AMERICAN PYRAMID

Travel almost 1,000 miles north-east of Taos and set your GPS at 38°39'37.55" N 90°03'43.66" W the enquiring dowser will be high on the top of Monks Mound near East St. Louis, Illinois. The pyramidologists will tell you that of all the ancient civilizations in North America human hands have built no greater earthwork.

Standing about a mile from the great Mississippi River the monument is 92 feet tall, 950 feet in length and 835 feet wide. The base covers about 14.4 acres and possesses a volume of about 21.5 million cubic feet. Experts say it was built with non-local soil, limestone blocks, along with bald cypress and red cedar posts. The limestone indicates a construction period between 3,000 to 1,000 BCE.

Known as the Cahokia Mounds the community at its peak contained about 20,000 people. The trading area covered most of the Plains and even beyond. Betty Lou and I visited Cahokia in the fall of 2011 and reported on our visit there in HOLY DIRT, SACRED EARTH.

Is it part of the Cosmic Principle? There is a "Yes" and a "No" and it is up for debate and perhaps time. On the surface there is nothing that resembles a pyramid but according to Dr. Timothy R. Pauketat, archaeologist and professor of anthropology at the University of Illinois there is a distinct possibility. In his book *Cahokia : Ancient Americas Great City on the Mississippi* he writes: "Cahokia was so large-covering three to five square miles-that archaeologists have yet to probe many portions of it. Its centerpiece was an open fifty-acre Grand Plaza, surrounded by packed-clay pyramids. The size of thirty-five football fields, the Grand Plaza was at the time the biggest public space ever conceived and executed north of Mexico."

So time and digs will tell. The Cahokia Indians considered the place holy ground and from an energy point of view it certainly packs a wallop. There are three leys passing through the complex forming the letter H.

At Monks Mound one ley runs north-west to south-east and the other runs east-west. Both leys at Monks Mound are strong and triple-haired and by all logic, a pyramid reflecting the Cosmic Principle should be standing there. The exact crossing point occurs at the top of the Mound where the path splits. Coordinates: 38°39′37.47" N 90°03′43.62" W

On the west side of the Mound not so deep underground there is a blind spring which produces a nest of at least 13 geospirals, one of which has 49 rings.

The east-west ley leaves the Mound and parallels the Collinsville Road a short distance to the famous Woodhenge which was part of the

Cahokia culture. The ley runs through the exact center of the ancient site while another north-west ley running south-east traverses the site. Both cross a few inches off the center post at 38°39′35.70″ N 90°04′30.15″ W.

Here there is another blind spring which may be connected to the one at Monks Mound. One thing is very positive: another nest of geospirals radiating Yin healing and relaxing energy. When you visit be sure to take a blanket and quietly relax for twenty minutes, seated or lying down inside the Woodhenge Circle. You will be glad you did.

If you feel some spirits moving around or even observing your prone condition say "Hello". They are likely to be the Cahokia Guardians — spirits of shamans still on duty some eight centuries after community closed down.

Even without a Cosmic Principle, the Cahokia site is a powerful vortex, closely comparable to Sedona, Glastonbury, Ararat and Giza. There are many ancient mounds dotting the American landscape but none possesses the complete Principle, physically or in phantom terms. Still, they are all sacred and we respect that.

# THE SACRED CITY OF CARAL IN PERU

The City of Caral was a large settlement in the Supe Valley, Barranca province, Peru, some 120 miles north of Lima. As it remains, Caral is the most ancient urban city in all of the Americas and it contains the remains of pyramids.

Excavators have described the city as pre-ceramic and at least 6,000 years old. It was a thriving metropolis about the same time as the general run of pyramids were being built in Egypt. The complex is spread out over 150 acres and contains plazas, temples and residential buildings.

Discovered by Paul Kosok in 1948 it received little attention because it lacked many typical artifacts that were archaeologically acceptable throughout the Andes at the time.

However, it presents several fascinating points: One, no trace of warfare has been found at Caral: no battlements, no weapons, no mutilated bodies. Archaeologist Ruth Shady who worked extensively in the area said findings suggest it was a gentle society, built on commerce and pleasure. In one of the temples, they uncovered 32 flutes made of condor and pelican bones and 37 cornets of deer and llama bones.

Another point: There are 19 temple complexes at Caral and the main one is known as Templo Mayor. Construction date is unknown. The Pacific coast is a mere 12 miles away and so storms and time have taken their toll on this ancient community, consequently it is difficult to ascertain if any of the buildings possessed apexes.

However, if one dowses the remains of this sacred place, the pendulum insists on swinging counter-clockwise only on one of the pyramid relics. It is called Piramide Menor or Minor Pyramid. Archaeologists should rest assured the Cosmic Principle works at Caral in South America. Bernard suggests it is over 7,000 years old. Incidentally, the Sacred City of Caral is a UNESCO World Heritage Center and their website contains a video of the ancient place. Dowsers can find it at coordinates: 10°58′30.49" S 77°31′12.68" W

# PHARAOHS STILL LIVE IN THE WEST

The Cosmic Principle exists in many ways principally with the major pyramids but also with monuments that are scattered across cities of the western world. That is the Egyptian obelisk and you will find them in Rome, Paris, London and New York. There are also great imitations standing around. Still, when it comes to obelisk design the Egyptians were late-comers. Monolithic stones towering up to the heavens have been around for more than 15,000 years. Some call them menhirs, others standing stones. In many cases the ancient people discovered that if they talked to a tall stone good harvests and healthy living would occur. James Michener describes this function very well in his book *The Source*. In Britain standing stones were used frequently to mark ancient ley lines.

The coming of the pharaohs saw the development of the obelisks as we know them. The true Egyptian obelisk was created from a single block of red granite. The flat surfaces were covered with hieroglyphs expressing prayers and salutations to the gods and listing the accomplishments of a pharaoh. Each obelisk was capped with a small pyramid sheathed in gold or electrum, an alloy of gold and silver, to reflect the dazzling rays of the sun god Ra. Nevertheless, true obelisks reflecting Cosmic Principle always contain a pointed apex with four sides meeting at a point. Without the critical plan, an obelisk does not reflect the energy.

Many of the 21 known ancient Egyptian obelisks have been sold, hijacked or confiscated leaving Egypt itself with only five. Incredibly Rome has 13, all carted away from the land of the pharaohs in the days of the Empire. The rest are spread across the western hemisphere from Istanbul to New York City.

Three of them are named Cleopatra's Needle. It's a popular nickname but totally inappropriate as we shall see. However they are all capped with mini-pyramids

"Cleopatra's Needle" is a 200 year-old public relations gimmick that seized the imagination of the crowds. In reality the needles had nothing to do with the ill-fated Egyptian queen but general publicity still seems to retain the falsehood. Catchy PR gimmicks die slowly.

Three ancient obelisks were transported west in the 19<sup>th</sup> century and erected in London, Paris and New York City. The obelisks in London and New York are a pair and the one in Paris is also part of a pair originally from a different site in Luxor, where its twin still remains.

As dowsers, we need to take a look at the fate of the obelisks because each radiates the energies of the Cosmic Principle and the interesting aspect of each one is that anyone armed with a simple pendulum can stand and measure the energies at quite large distances from each monument.

# A POWER PYRAMID IN PARIS

For dowsers, a great place to swing a pendulum is in the very heart of Paris where there is a very odd situation in the Cosmic Principle: a modern pyramid and an ancient obelisk both standing on two impressive leys.

The modern pyramid is to be found at the entrance to The Louvre or Musée du Louvre which is one of the world's largest museums and also a historic monument in Paris. The museum which has been a great landmark since 1792 stands on the Right Bank of the River Seine.

While the Museum is old the pyramid is a modern addition. Completed in 1989 it is stunning, attractive and ultramodern because it consists of 673 panes of glass supported by metal frames. It stands 71 feet tall, contains a square base with four sides, each measuring 115 feet. It is the doorway to the great Louvre.

Why?

The pyramid with an underground lobby existing beneath it, came about because of problems stemming from the Louvre's main entrance. The heavily worn gateway could not handle the enormous numbers of daily visitors so an underground bypass had to be created. Present day visitors entering through the pyramid descend into a spacious lobby then re-ascend into the main buildings. What an excellent bypass!

It was the brainchild of Chinese American architect I. M. Pei. If you have visited the Rock and Roll Hall of Fame in Cleveland or the East Building of the National Gallery of Art in Washington or Place Ville Marie in Montreal, you will have viewed some of his work.

Now back to dowsing.

First and foremost the Louvre pyramid fits the Cosmic Principle. Its Area of Influence reaches about two miles in any direction which means a counter-clockwise spin. Underneath there is a large blind spring manifesting a bundle of relaxing geospirals, all of which require mapping.

This is a great place to hang out if you wish to soak up this powerful Yin energy, find a place to meditate or snooze and if a gendarme does not tell you to move on, you will enjoy the experience.

For energy seekers, there is more. Two triple-haired leys cross both the pyramid and the museum. One comes down Avenue de la Opera after passing through the Opera House.

The other comes from the east, passes through the Louvre and its Pyramid, then passes through the historic Garden of the Tuileries, created by Catherine de Medicis in 1564, through the Place de la Concorde, then along the Avenue of the Champs-Elysees, before crossing the Place de Charles de Gaulle with its famous Arc de Triomphe. It does not stop there but goes on along the Avenue de la Grande Armée.

The distance between the Louvre and the Arc de Triomphe is about two miles and the ley is flanked by numerous geospirals which is one good reason why the official Tourism Books say the Garden of the Tuileries is a great place to promenade and relax.

And you may have wondered why so many people of all nations come and just hang out in this wonderful place. Many years ago, 1983 in fact, when I wandered along this very route with a lady called Myra, a French soldier on leave from Algeria told us "Il est le paradis sur terre!" which meant "It is Heaven on Earth." We could all feel the Yin energy of the place, but that was not all. There is more.

# THE OBELISK ON A LEY

It is at the Place de la Concorde that ancient Egypt makes its presence felt on this ley. The Egyptian needle is properly called Obélisque de Louxor because it used to stand at the entrance to the Temple at Luxor.

This yellow granite column stands 75 feet tall and weighs over 250 tons. Decorated with hieroglyphics it exalts the reign of Ramses II (1279 to 1213 BCE). During his long 67 year reign, he had many wives who bore him 111 sons and 51 daughters. He also became known as a great military leader, conducted extensive building programs and was responsible for some colossal statues and obelisks.

The Luxor obelisk was gifted to France by Muhammed Ali, Khedive of Egypt. How the French picked it up from Luxor is another story. The French government ordered a specially built seagoing lighter — a flat bottomed barge — from the Toulon naval yard. The 160 feet long, flat bottomed, three masted ship was named the Louqsor and it sailed 540 miles up the River Nile to Luxor where 300 workers had dug a canal so that the ship could dock next to the obelisk.

Using a complicated set of blocks and tackles, yarda:
the obelisk was carefully lowered to a horizontal positi(
tioned on the ship along with its original pedestal.

The ships departed Egypt on April 1ˢᵗ 1833 and reꭤ.... ꭒ..... ꭒ.... ꭒ
in mid-August. The re-erection of the obelisk at the center of the Place
de la Concorde took place in October 1836 at a ceremony orchestrated
by King Louis Philippe. It is flanked on both sides by fountains that were
constructed at the same time.

Did anyone notice that the capstone, the pyramidion that gave the
needle its power was missing? It was believed stolen sometime in the 6ᵗʰ
century BCE. The French government remedied the situation by adding
a gold-leafed pyramid cap to the top of the obelisk in 1998, some 162
years after it graced the Paris scene.

The French authorities refused to use the obelisk's original pedestal
because it included the statues of sixteen fully sexed baboons and was
therefore too obscene for public exhibition — this, after 3,000 years on
show in Egypt. The current pedestal shows drawn illustrations of the
complicated machinery used in transporting the Egyptian relic.

Is it a coincidence that the obelisk came from a ley line in Egypt and
now stands on a ley in modern Paris? Whoever designed Paris understood
and worked with Earth energies to create a city with its key avenues and
attractions on two major leys, including the Pyramid of the Louvre. As
the French would say with a shrug: "Bien entendu, il est tout simplement
une coïncidence." Of course, it is just a coincidence. What else ?

There is a postscript to the whole affair. The Khedive of Egypt originally gifted two of the Ramses obelisks but the second one was found
too dangerous to move, so it remains today standing and complete with
its capstone at the Temple of Luxor. It was officially gifted back to Egypt
by French President Francois Mitterrand in the early 1990s.

## NOTE FOR DOWSERS:

Paris Coordinates:
The Louvre Pyramid: 48°51′39.47" N 2°20′09.29" W
The Luxor Obelisk: 48°51′55.68" N 2°19′16.15" E

Both are on the same ley.

The blind spring and its geospirals require mapping.

# LONDON'S "CLEOPATRA" NEEDLE.

I f you're going to fight a battle, make sure you have energy in addition to cannons and men. Rear Admiral Horatio Nelson and the Royal Navy did just that when they ousted Napoleon and his Grand Armée from Egypt. One was the Battle of the Nile which took place in Abukir Bay in 1798 and the other was the Battle of Alexandria in 1801 — both places have renowned leys.

In appreciation Muhammed Ali, the khedive or king of Egypt gave one of the Alexandria obelisks to the United Kingdom as a gift of appreciation. That was in 1819. It was a great honor but the British government, suffering economically, socially and politically and consequently strapped for cash, just could not afford to transport the 224 ton block of granite to England. The gift sat in Alexandria for over half a century.

Finally a doctor, surgeon and dermatologist, William James Erasmus Wilson decided to pay for the shipping. Not only that he took over and organized the entire mission to collect the gift.

The obelisk transporter was strange and had a name that belied its origin. Nicknamed "The Cleopatra" it consisted of an iron cylinder which contained a bow and stern with the giant obelisk inside. Equipped with a rudder this monster or pontoon as it was called, was towed like a barge by a ship named The Olga.

The obelisk departed Alexandria on September 21st 1877 and all went well until the mission came to the temperamental Bay of Biscay, north of Spain. On October 14th an Atlantic storm struck the ship. The iron cylinder with its precious cargo broke loose and started to tilt precariously. In a gallant but tragic attempt to rescue The Cleopatra, six crewmen from The Olga were sent into the raging seas. They were all lost. The remaining crew on the sinking Olga, the captain and five men were saved.

Incredibly, Fate and the elements did not allow the iron cylinder with its historic cargo to sink. A few days later it was discovered drifting, promptly retrieved and towed to Ferrol in north-west Spain.

A paddle tugboat named The Anglia arrived and successfully towed the cylinder to Gravesend on the River Thames in England. It arrived on January 21st 1878 and on September 12th that year, the so called Cleopatra's Needle was erected on the Victoria Embankment, London. The gift to Britain had taken 59 years to reach its destination. William Erasmus Wilson was knighted by Queen Victoria in 1881. The names of the six crewmen who died on the mission are engraved on a plaque on the pedestal.

There are two impressive sphinxes guarding this relic of old Egypt and a single ley passes across the eastern sphinx on a north-south route. Perhaps curiously, perhaps not, the ley passes through the Library and Museum of Freemasonry before coming south to the Needle. It then traverses the Thames and cuts through Lambeth Palace which for 800 years has been the London residence of the Archbishop of Canterbury. The area of Influence of this Egyptian needle is over one mile.

FOR DOWSERS: Coordinates: 51°30'30.61" N 0°07'13.08" W.

Suggestion: Hold a pendulum by its chain, stand on Waterloo Bridge where you can look down on the Victoria Embankment, focus on the so-called Cleopatra's Needle and watch the pendulum swing counter-clockwise. A Cosmic Principle! Enjoy!

# THE THIRD OBELISK: NEW YORK CITY

This ancient piece of man-carved red granite stands majestically in New York's Central Park. It is 3,500 years old, 69 feet tall, weighs 220 tons and as the New York Post noted recently many New Yorkers do not know it exists.

This great antique, also misnamed Cleopatra's Needle, nestles in the trees opposite the Metropolitan Museum of Art. The nearest ley is a few yards away near the Museum but that does not hamper this relic of ancient Egypt from radiating its own Cosmic energy. With its four-sided and pointed apex or cornerstone it has an Area of Influence over a large section of Central Park.

As with the Paris and London obelisks, the New York monument is the handiwork of Thutmose the Third, the warrior Pharaoh who is buried in one of the most prestigious tombs in the Valley of the Kings near Luxor and Karnak. His sideline specialty during his 54 year reign seems to have been creating obelisks and like the others, it too has a strange story of how it reached East 81$^{st}$ Street in New York City.

It too had its main existence at Heliopolis, the City of the Sun, once the spiritual center for sun worship in ancient Egypt. It survived the Persian and Alexandrian invasions before the Romans in AD moved it to Alexandria on the Mediterranean coast. The towering monuments were placed in the Caesarium, a temple named in honor of Julius Caesar.

Although the temple had been built during Cleopatra's reign, the obelisks arrived there some 15 years after she had committed suicide.

The United States was the only western power not to send a representative to Egypt for the lavish and spectacular opening of the Suez Canal organized by the Khedive Ishmail in 1869. One reason may have been the US was recovering from a brutal and costly civil war, another was the fact France did not want the US to be invited.

However, in 1878 when visiting Americans saw the London obelisk a general cry went up –"we want one in America." The media picked up on the chorus. William Hulbert, editor of the New York World newspaper and Elbert E. Farman who was US Consul-General in Cairo launched a public campaign to obtain one. The Khedive, strapped for funds, finally agreed after various rounds of talks on condition the obelisk would be mounted in New York City. A clause in the contract enabled Egyptian Authorities to reclaim the obelisk if it was no longer wanted or treated badly. Wise thinking.

In fact in 2011 in a letter to the City Mayor Michael Bloomberg, famous archaeologist Zahi Hawass, secretary-general for Egypt's Supreme Council of Antiquities vigorously complained that the New York obelisk was "severely weathered over the past years" adding "no efforts have been made to conserve it." He said he had received photographs showing "severe damage" particularly to the hieroglyphic texts which in places have been "completely worn away."

The letter triggered a rebuttal from the Parks Department and Central Park Conservancy which pointed out the obelisk's damage was caused by being embedded in desert sands centuries before.

Still, The Conservancy brought in an Illinois-based expert conservationist Bartosz Dajnowski to clean the obelisk with lasers and then repair cracks before covering it with a protective coating. The results are said to bring improved hieroglyphics and preserve the obelisk for many future years.

Meanwhile back to Egypt. The Khedive finally approved the sale and William Vanderbilt the railroad magnate covered the transportation of the obelisk from Alexandria to New York. The man chosen for the task was Henry Gorringe a decorated Navy commander.

On October 16, 1879, with the assistance of 100 Arabs, Gorringe packed the obelisk into an 83 feet long crate then loaded it into the hold of the Egyptian ship SS Dessoug. It took almost a month to reach New York and the Hudson River. A special railroad track was built and for five months laborers inched the monument along aided by roll boxes and a pile-driver engine to move the obelisk to Central Park where it arrived January 22nd 1881. Gorringe received a hero's welcome but strangely he died four years later from injuries sustained while hopping a train in Philadelphia. The monument over his last resting place is an exact scale model of the obelisk that he transported from Egypt. Like any perfect obelisk with an apex it fits into the Cosmic Principle and radiates peaceful relaxing energy from a grave site.

Back at the obelisk thousands turned out to watch as the ancient monument was mounted on a pedestal at Central Park's Graywacke Knoll. A time capsule was buried on the site. It contained a copy of the

1870 United States census, the Bible, Webster's Dictionary, the complete works of William Shakespeare, a guide to Egypt and a facsimile of the Declaration of Independence.

The New York Post in an article says that as the cornerstone was laid at least 9,000 Freemasons marched up Fifth Avenue to commemorate the ceremony.

FOR DOWSERS: Thomas Campbell, the Director of the Metropolitan Museum of Art which is across the road, says the best time to visit the so-called Cleopatra's Needle is in the spring when the obelisk is surrounded by flowing magnolias and crabapple trees.

A TURKISH DELIGHT — A WELL TRAVELED OBELISK

If your travels take you to Istanbul, Turkey, hire a cab to Sultan Ahmet Parki and you will find not one, but two obelisks separated only by a short walk.

It's not on any ley but it does have a capstone matching the Cosmic Principle and of course, pendulums in the vicinity swing counter-clockwise.

The obelisk was first created by Thutmose III who was the warrior pharaoh of Egypt's 18th and largest dynasty. Thutmose who lived some 14 centuries BCE set up the obelisk in the seventh gateway or pylon to the great temple at Karnak, about two miles from Luxor.

In 357 AD Constantine II had it and another obelisk transported by barge down the River Nile to Alexandria where it was erected to mark his being on the throne for twenty years. It remained there until 390 when Emperor Theodosius, the scourge of anything non-Christian, had it shipped to Constantinople and erected on the spina of the Roman Hippodrome. It then became the Obelisk of Theodosius.

Constantinople officially became Istanbul when the Republic of Turkey was created in 1923 and enforced nationally and internationally when the Turkish Postal Service Law came into effect in 1930. Constantinople was history.

FOR DOWSERS: It's on the Binbirdirek, Istanbul, Turkey. The old Hippodrome. A large blind spring needs tracking, plus a nest of geospirals. The obelisk coordinates are: 41°00′21.20" N 28°58′31.34" E

The second monument is known as the Walled Obelisk or the Constantine Obelisk. Reaching 105 feet (32 m) into the Turkish sky it is somewhat unique because it was constructed of roughly cut stones by Constantine VII.

Originally it was covered with gilded bronze plaques or plates that portrayed the victories of Basil I, the grandfather of Constantine. At one time someone mounted a sphere on the apex, however the ball and the plates were stolen and melted down during the sacking of Constantinople by the cash-strapped Fourth Crusade on its way to recapture Jerusalem.

It was damaged over the years by young soldiers climbing the monument but now much has been repaired. Today, the Constantine Obelisk sits on a sunken pedestal surrounded by a protective wall. It shows a pyramid apex and thereby forms a Cosmic Principle. There is plenty of room for dowsers to view this ancient monument.

FOR DOWSERS: It's on the Binbirdirek, Istanbul, Turkey. The old Hippodrome. The coordinates are: 41°00′18.69" N 28°58′ 30.55" E

# AN OBELISK IN THE HOLY CITY

One obelisk went to the Hippodrome in Turkey, the second obelisk from Thutmose's Karnak went to Rome where it was erected on the spina, the median of Circus Maximus in the fall of 357 AD.

There it stood until after the fall of the Western Roman Empire in the 5th century. Circus Maximus, the scene of so many chariot races and violence, was abandoned and statues and obelisks were eventually broken up or pulled down. Eventually Thutmose's obelisk was buried by mud and debris and almost forgotten.

It stayed lost throughout the 1,000 year Dark Ages until the 16th century when Pope Sixtus V ordered a search for the ancient monument. When found some 23 feet underground it was in three pieces. Experts put it together and on August 3, 1588, after more than a year of restoration the Egyptian obelisk made of red granite was raised in the Piazza San Giovanni in Laterano, where it still stands.

Today it is called the Lateran obelisk and is the largest free standing ancient Egyptian obelisk in the world standing 105.6 feet and 149.9 feet with its base. It is also the tallest obelisk in Italy with a weight of 455 tons.

Nobody mentions it much, but this monument stands on a major ley in the Holy City. One wonders what would happen if one popped round to the Holy Office and asked "Did you know there is a triple-haired ley....?" It is doubtful anyone would say more than "Ha! Ha! Solo una coincidenza."

If you are dowsing in Rome the obelisk can be found in the square across from the Archbasilica of St. John Lateran and the famous Lateran Palace. The obelisk has four sides and an apex and in spite of the fact that someone mounted a small cross on the cornerstone, the Cosmic Principle still operates. If a dowser stands anywhere in the Piazza and focuses on the obelisk the pendulum will still swing counter-clockwise.

The powerful three line ley line cuts through the obelisk. It comes through the ruins of the Roman Forum, the Temple of Antonino and Faustina, the west side of the famous Colosseum where it then passes along Via San Giovanni. Passing through the obelisk, it then cuts across the famous Lateran Palace. This is an ancient palace of the Roman Empire which later became the main papal residence in southeast Rome. The ley also touches the Archbasilica of St. John Lateran, the cathedral church of Rome.

There are other leys in Rome but only one runs through the Lateran Obelisk. Coordinates: 41°53′12.53″ N 12°30′17.27″ W

With a lot of geospirals in and around the square from a deep blind spring underground, plus the Cosmic Principle seated above the needle, it is an excellent spot for relaxation, meditation, photography and other healthy things in Modern Rome. Sit on the monument steps for a while and feel the Yin energy and if you feel like it, say a prayer of thanks to the Creator or whoever in the Cosmos you talk with.

# A GOLDEN PYRAMID IN ILLINOIS

Folks driving through Wadsworth, Illinois and finding themselves on North Dilleys Road may well think they have been transplanted into ancient Egypt. Because there stands a golden pyramid resplendent in all its glory amid an area that resembles the Giza Plateau.

This is the work of Jim Onan, a long time admirer of the Great Pyramid specifically and Egyptian culture generally. After building his own cement business, Jim along with wife Linda and family of five, found his attention drawn not only to pyramids but a university study that suggested the Giza pyramids generated some form of energy.

It was this curiosity that prompted the construction of several small pyramids close to his home. When visitors arrived and put their hands out, they felt strange sensations emanating from the tops of the pyramids.

To experiment on the latent energy he built a 13 foot pyramid. One of his sons studying botany at a university suggested that by placing some plants inside the monument they might grow better. The results were stunning. The plants grew three times as fast inside than outside the pyramid.

One day, Jim was talking with his wife Linda about what kind of home they should build and Linda jokingly said "Why don't you build it out of a pyramid?" It was a great idea and so he built a Pyramid home for his family and it was an exact replica model of the Great Pyramid at Giza but one ninth the size and with a pool.

As the building took shape a strange phenomenon occurred. Spring water started bubbling up and flooded the ground floor. Plans for an indoor pool were scrapped and experts were brought in to channel the water into the surrounding area.

It appears the Onan family had tapped into a blind spring sitting deep below their property and an outlet had occurred. Still very enthused about pyramidology, Jim Onan decided to coat the pyramid with gold. One million dollars and the pyramid was coated with 24-karat gold making it the largest gold plated structure in North America.

Immediately it became a media and tourist sensation. Visitors came by the thousands. So did Michael Jackson who wanted to shoot a music video there. Then one day, a worker on the pyramid tasted the water, found it potable — and more, so he drank it every day and shortly after claimed his blood pressure was back to normal. Others started to drink the spring water and many claimed to feel better or to have certain ailments cured. Critics suggested it might be a placebo effect but others who felt the energy knew it was something different.

Yes, it is a true pyramid and matches the Cosmic Principle. Pendulum people will find a strong counter-clockwise rotation either in person on location or by using Google Earth.

From a dowsing viewpoint, the Golden Pyramid at Wadsworth IL actually stands on a single line ley that runs north-east to south-west. It comes out of Lake Michigan at the Winthrop Harbor Yacht Club and crosses Wadsworth Village before coming to the Golden Pyramid site. A second ley can be found on Highway 15 heading towards Chicago.

The abundance of water at the site comes from a large blind spring that exists on the west part of the complex which in turn prompts eleven geospirals, one of which is a 49-ring manifestation. All combined, the energy generated there is extremely relaxing, a very healthy Yin exposure and a good place to conduct a health spa.

NOTES FOR DOWSERS: The address is 37921 N Dilleys Rd, Wadsworth, IL It is about 50 miles north of Chicago. Coordinates: 42°24′47.91″ N 87°56′27.83″ W.

Check: A second ley running along N. Dilleys Road (Highway 15) right by the entrance to the Golden Pyramid. It appears to connect West Milwaukee in the north with Chicago's O'Hare International Airport Terminal in the south.

# A MODERN PYRAMID IN LAS VEGAS

Pilgrims to Las Vegas, Nevada since October 1993 may have encountered the Luxor Las Vegas. It is a 30-storey hotel named after the city of Luxor known to the ancient Egyptians as Thebes.

Shaped in true pyramid style it even picks up on old Babylonian architecture with twin 22-storey ziggurat towers. Ziggurat?

A ziggurat is a 4,000 year old method of building a temple in the form of a terraced pyramid with successively receding stories. The resort owned by MGM Resorts International has over 4,400 rooms along with over 2,000 slot machines and 87 tables for gaming.

Occasionally big corporations do good things. In 2010 the Luxor in Las Vegas had a 4 Key rating from the Green Key Eco-Rating Program which evaluates "sustainable" hotel operations.

For dowsers too the pyramid is built in true Great Pyramid style and when you go with your pendulum, it only swings counter-clockwise. The Luxor Pyramid's Area of Influence is substantial too. For instance for flyers, when you get off your aircraft at McCarran International Airport, hold a pendulum in true dowsing search style and focus on Luxor Pyramid. Then watch what happens. Pyramid Power! Or better still, the Luxor reflects the true Cosmic Principle. Caution! In your enthusiasm do not enter this or any other casino with a swinging pendulum. Management really gets bent out of shape.

# THE EL DORADO-VEGAS-NELLIS LEY

There's no ley running through the Luxor in Vegas, however a major ley does cross Lake Las Vegas. On a north-north-west course it appears in the silver and gold rich El Dorado Canyon area, specifically crossing Highway 165 east of the Nelson Ghost Town. It heads over the mountains to Boulder City and crosses the Nevada Way/Wyoming intersection, then touches Reflection Bay on Lake Las Vegas before heading across the eastern side of Nellis Air Force Base.

FOR DOWSERS:
El D Canyon, Highway 165 E 35°42´34.75" N 00114°48´13.97" W
East side Nellis AFB: 36°14´48.04" N 114°56´44.98" W.
More work needs to be done on this ley.

# ESSAY: TIME OUT — EXPLORING THE COSMIC PRINCIPLE

For years I enjoyed being a newspaper journalist and news photographer. For some more years while working in radio I enjoyed producing explorative documentaries — finding out stuff. Now I'm a dowser exploring the effects of Earth energies.

It is truly fascinating to hear from our spirit friends, notably Bernard and others, that the Great Pyramid at Giza was built to a Cosmic Principle, a formula so simple that using it generates an energy that spins a human held pendulum counter-clockwise.

Then we discover that it is not the pyramid itself that generates the energy but the plan, the formula, the square complete with a diagonal cross that touches each of the four corners.

This brings about another revelation. Both the pyramid and the drawn plan produce large Areas of Influence that generate pendulums to spin counter-clockwise.

AS we have seen when a pendulum is held by hand over or near a Cosmic Principle the instrument starts to rotate so fast that the human hand becomes incapable of holding the chain or string connector.

Could it be that one day science will create an energy sensor along with a mechanical method of holding a pendulum so that no matter how fast the unit spins this energy can be used utilized? In other words: Is the Cosmic Principle a generator? Also is it near to Perpetual Motion? One wonders.

The human body is a generator of energy and it is reflected in auras that exist around all living things, humans, animals, trees and plants. After the sun has just gone down over the horizon, find a solitary tree and position yourself so you can see it silhouetted. After a few moments you will witness a shimmering almost as big again as the tree. That is the tree's aura, an energy field.

A pair of L-rods searching for the edge of an aura on a living being will cross when it reaches the outer limits. One can do the same thing with a pendulum.

But this is where things change. Hold a pendulum over a man or boy's head and the pendulum will swing clockwise. Do the same with a woman or a girl and the pendulum will swing counter-clockwise. Does this make females cosmic? I have no idea. It just happens.

As mentioned earlier, hold a pendulum over different human fingers and each finger is different from the other — either clockwise or counter-clockwise.

We mentioned earlier that anything counter-clockwise is Yin. A yin energy is distinctly feminine in nature, it is also quiet and passive, encourages intuiting, encourages right-brain activity which promotes creativity and inventiveness. Yin is also compassionate.

It is all very well to recognize a Yin consciousness in living things in Nature, because as most people know there is an opposite known as Yang. This is Universal Law. For every positive there must be a negative and vice versa. But how about inanimate objects? When a pendulum swings counter-clockwise over a pyramid where or what is the opposite?

Pyramids and obelisks with pyramidion tops are Yin. So could there be something else that manifests the Cosmic Principle's force to induce a pendulum to swing counter-clockwise?

These are simple experiments that any dowser can enjoy exploring and questioning. Often the answers trigger new questions.

Write the numbers one to nine on a piece of paper, leaving a small space between each. Thus 1 2 3 4 5 6 7 8 9.

Hold a pendulum over each number ranging from one to eight and the pendulum will freely swing clockwise. Hold it over number nine presented as a 9 and it insists on swinging counter-clockwise. In fact, the swing is similar to a pendulum held over a pyramid. It gathers momentum to the point of breaking. Incidentally, hold it over the written word "nine" and the swing is clockwise.

We are not finished: Nine has long been known as a Cosmic number because of its power in mathematics and physics. Look at the Cosmic Principle on paper, the roughly drawn square with a diagonal cross. There are eight 45 degree angles and each one of those 45s reduces to nine. There are eight 90 degree angles and each one reduces to a nine. The four center angles each 90 degrees equals four times 90 is 360 degrees. That reduces to the cosmic nine. The plan of the Cosmic Principle is a nine. Each true pyramid contains the magical number nine.

During our research we discovered a photograph of a clay tablet from the 45,000 pieces in the Yale Babylonian Collection. It is known as YBC 7289. The photo was taken by Bill Hasselman of the Mathematics Department, University of British Columbia. The tablet displays a set of cuneiform numbers equating to the square root of 2. Fascinating stuff in mathematics. However the interesting point for dowsers is that the numbers are set in a square with a diagonal cross — a Cosmic Principal! Yes, a pendulum swings counter-clockwise when held over the tablet. Positive indications the Sumerian graphologists knew all about the Principal 6,000 years ago.

# EXPANDING THE SEARCH

Once one starts tooling or researching a subject bits and pieces pertinent to the search start appearing as if by magic. Some people, mainly of a skeptical urge, may argue it is pure coincidence but I am inclined to think the message flies out or is broadcast on the ether and people consciously or subconsciously are attracted to the energy and pick it up. Human mental energies are much more powerful than than they get credited for, particularly by their owners.

Christmas came and some kind friends gifted us a small jar of Cypriot Pyramid Salt. It was a curiosity because somewhere in my distant past I served many years as a journalist, broadcaster and news photographer on the Mediterranean island of Cyprus. In all that time I never heard of Cypriot Pyramid Salt. So here it was, a product of Cyprus, packed in South Africa and sold by Trader Joe's in New Jersey.

Apparently it is a favorite in gourmet dining but the intriguing thing is — the salt crystals are actually shaped as pyramids. On average a crystal is about a quarter of an inch in size — and yes! The Pendulum insists on swinging counter-clockwise.

Pyramids are natural conveyors of the Cosmic Principle but there are others not so obvious. Back in 1991 my cruise travels took me to wander among the vendors who flock the harbor side at Acapulco on Mexico's Pacific Coast. A stamped .925 silver signet ring caught my eye because it carried a fine etching of the sacred Aztec Sun Calendar.

The original calendar also known as the famous Sun Stone or Stone of the Five Eras is a late post-classic Mexican sculpture. It rests in the National Anthropology Museum in Mexico City, weighs about 24 tons, is almost 12 feet in diameter and stands over three feet thick. With the coming of the Spanish, the stone was buried in the main square, el Zócalo in Mexico City.

Rediscovered just before Christmas in 1790 it was mounted on an exterior wall of the Cathedral, where it remained for almost a hundred years. Many scholars estimate the stone was carved between 1502 and 1521 making it about 500 years old. Others believe it is much older.

My silver signet ring with the stone embossed was perched on a display box on my desk. It caught my attention and as I picked it up Bernard's soft but articulate voice came through.

"Another piece of the puzzle. Use your pendulum," he said.

No ifs, ands or buts. It was a direct order. I stared at the strange face and the markings as I had many times before, but this time was different.

"There's no pyramid, not even a square. Your Cosmic Principle does not fit," I claimed, sensing I was about to be shot down.

"Use your pendulum."

Moments later a pendulum was suspended over the top of the silver ring. Sure enough it started swinging — counter-clockwise!

This immediately created concern in my mind. There was nothing that resembled a pyramid or a square with a diagonal cross. Hurriedly

I browsed over to the National Museum of Mexico, downloaded and printed a large photo of the famous stone

The pendulum immediately swung counter-clockwise.

A magnifying glass was brought in. Suddenly among all the circular images my eyes caught sight of four markers.

An article on the internet suggested a possible geographic significance. The four points might relate to the four corners of the earth or the cardinal points. If this were true then the four points would constitute a square and the four points joined in a diagonal cross would complete the design.

"See!" Bernard's voice was edged with a touch of triumph.

"No, I do not really see. It appears the Cosmic Principle can be embedded in an ancient calendar that's well over 500 years old," I replied. "So we are back to the old question: how did the designers of the sun calendar know about this? Who told them the Earth had four corners? The Church says..."

"Our friends the Sumerians knew this when their scribes wrote all about Earth in clay tablets over 6,000 years ago," said Bernard easily.

"But there's no diagonal cross on the stone," I protested.

"Isn't there?" The voice was edged with an easy mockery. "Just because your eyes cannot see, does not mean it fails to exist. Your higher consciousness together with a pendulum shows it is there, plain and simple."

"Phantom?"

"Not a bit. You simply cannot see it," he noted quickly. "There are many things in your Universe that you use but are not aware."

"For instance?"

"Betty Lou, how many times has she played the piano."

"Thousands. Countless times."

"Does she know there is a Cosmic note among the keys?"

I wanted to brand the idea as ridiculous, then I recalled that some musical gurus once claimed that F sharp was Cosmic. Bernard read my thought.

"Those are sounds. This is a note," he said simply.

Moments later I sat at the piano and followed his instructions. "Hold your pendulum and let it swing clockwise and play any note except a middle C."

I played all the notes except the middle C and the pendulum happily swung clockwise.

"Now play the C several times for a continual note."

Instantly, the pendulum reacted with a rapid change to a counter-clockwise spin.

"Does this work with any C?" The question was frivolous, of course any C note would react the same way. "So why the C note, Bernard?"

A brief sigh came over the Etheric. "The C note is pure. It's the only note in music where there are no sharps or flats. All music theory is based on the C note. It has a frequency of 432 Herz and a Herz is a unit of frequency of one cycle per second of your time. It abbreviates to 432 Hz."

"Four thirty-two reduces to nine," I said with a nod trying hard to keep up.

"Smart chappie!" commented Bernard in that dry English voice. "432 hz, is a cosmic frequency known throughout all the Cosmos. It resonates with all Nature including you. It is a natural healer and to a listener it brings warm feelings of peace and well-being. If you encounter rocks on the road of life, music that is based or tuned to 432 Hz will clear them. Such music also expands the human consciousness and makes humans more intuitive."

This raises the question: "Is the lonely C note a part of the Cosmic Principle, and if it is — why? Bernard did not reply. He had gone leaving me to my own questions and hopefully answers.

Now, here's a thing: If you keep striking a C note and have someone holding a pendulum walk away from the keyboard, the pendulum will continue to spin counter-clockwise. Does this mean there is an Area of Influence, and if so, how far does it go. We have not explored that yet.

So much depends on the magical number nine. The plan of the Cosmic Principle is a nine, the C note tone reduces to nine. Bernard referred to all this as a puzzle. Puzzle for what? For many days wherever I went, whatever ideas crossed my mind, I would test them with a pendulum for the counter-clockwise effect.

There are seven colors generally accepted in metaphysics, chakra specialists and people who watch rainbows. They are red, orange, yellow, green, blue, indigo and violet. For our various healing activities we keep a set of colored cloths in these colors.

The pendulum swung clockwise on all but one. Yellow. It swung vigorously counter-clockwise.

"Why? Bernard, are you listening?" No reply. In the closet I found some white, blue and yellow shirts. Same again. The yellow one caused a counter-clockwise spin.

Now, here's a thing. Look at the paragraph above where it lists the seven colors. Hold a pendulum in your right hand and with the pointing finger of the left hand (vice versa if left handed) go through each of the colors listed. Even when yellow is printed in black it triggers a counter-clockwise rotation. Therefore is it the color that generates a counter-clockwise spin or is it the printed word yellow?

This prompted more thought. Pendulums have always been a "free thinking" modality with the option to express answers four ways: clockwise, counter-clockwise, forward and back and side to side. For years and years the pendulum as part of the human psyche, the human consciousness has been able to answer questions for dowsers and all the other questers seeking information for themselves or clients.

But according to these findings, if the subject involves colors and yellow is involved, it will always generate a counter-clockwise swing which may not be the correct answer.

Example: If the pendulumist routinely expects a counter-clockwise swing to mean "No" asks the question is: "Is yellow good for me now?" The answer could be wrong.

Another oddity: the color yellow is an English word. In Spanish it is amarillo and in Italian giallo. Both words produce a counter-clockwise spin. It is the same in other languages such as Greek and traditional Chinese. The question now must rest with: Is it the intent or mention of the color that triggers a counter-clockwise spin?

The fact that the pendulum swings counter-clockkwise on some words only triggers more questions. It is a phenomenon that becomes increasingly difficult to understand as research expands.

We tested various words — physics, truth, prayer, ley line, geospiral, dynamite, Babylon, Egypt and Moses — all swung clockwise. When we tried the word Spirit the pendulum swung clockwise, but when the word was changed to Spiritual the pendulum swung counter-clockwise. Go figure!

It also spun counter-clockwise on two Biblical figures, Abraham and Job and a Book of Mormon prophet named Zenock. Other words that triggered counter-clockwise reaction included pyramid, cosmic principle, sacred and some different words below.

One day in early 2016 Betty Lou and I tracked leys through Princeton, New Jersey and found ourselves standing outside the Institute for Advanced Studies where Albert Einstein called home for a whole lot of years. Next day while studying photographs Betty Lou had taken, Bernard suddenly came through.

"Einstein! The elements! Have you tried those?"

"All our tests have been random. They don't make sense. There's no direction," I replied.

"Ah, try the list of elements, laddie."

On the internet at Jefferson Lab one can find a neat presentation of Periodic Table of Elements Listed by Atomic Number. Armed with a pendulum I dowsed each of the 118. Most produced a clockwise response — but eight produced a counter-clockwise spin.

They are: 40: ZIRCONIUM used in nuclear reactors; 65: TERBIUM a member of Rare Earth elements; 68: ERBIUM used in nuclear reactor rods and lasers; 74: TUNGSTEN has the highest melting point of any metal; 93: NEPTUNIUM used to produce Plutonium 238, also used for spacecraft generators and terrestrial navigation beacons; 99: EINSTEINIUM named after A. Einstein / radio-active, it was discovered in debris of the first hydrogen bomb; 102: NOBELIUM toxic due to radio activity. Discovered 1957. Plus 117: UNUNSEPTIUM super heavy artificial chemical element with unknown uses. In Physics it is known as the Island of Stability.

Dowsers with pendulums: put a finger on each Element and check it out for yourselves.

Again, the question: Why? There is a deep desire within that says this whole phenomenon of pendulum and words needs to be studied clinically to find — what? More questions.

Why some words react counter-clockwise and what do they mean? The Random House Webster's College Dictionary with its 1,500 plus pages contains a lot of words. Words starting with the letter A take up 99 pages ( that is another nine) so we scanned them with a pendulum. It swung counter-clockwise on the following:

Abacus, ábaco, abaque, Abakus, Agave, Antineutrino, Antipodes, Arsenal, Azimuth. Nine words!

Curiosity prompted us to take away the Anti from Neutrino. The result was still counter-clockwise. If some dedicated dowser wishes to scan the entire dictionary perhaps, just perhaps, there may be an interesting message waiting to be found.

Finally another riddle of words. There are particular words when standing alone trigger a counter-clockwise spin of the pendulum. But what about a collection of words?

Ever since the spiritual teacher the late Paul Solomon once suggested that the last part of the Lord's Prayer originated with ancient Egyptian mystics I have always wondered. Testing the Prayer everything swings clockwise until the pendulum reaches the words:

*"But deliver us from evil, For thine is the kingdom, The power and the glory, For ever and ever. Amen."*

Those entire words generate a counter-clockwise spin and that boggles the mind because it could mean entire books, like the pyramids are part of the Cosmic Principle.

As the reader may realize, I enjoy being a enquiring dowser always asking questions because I believe there is so much Earth energy that needs light — explorative light. Earth energy in its various manifestations is positively affecting people, cultures and business as we will now see in the notes ahead.

# BOOK FOUR

## TRACKING NORTH AMERICAN LEYS

While pyramids and obelisks can be awe inspiring, impressive, and conjure up visions of people through the ages and past events they can trigger all sorts of research and prompt many logical and far out illogical theories. In the case of the Great Pyramid of Giza the monument attracts 14 million visitors a year. But Giza is not alone. Pyramids and pyramidical shapes such as those found on the tops of the obelisks manifest energies that attract countless throngs of people every year.

One obvious element that must not be dismissed is the fact that the majority of pyramids and pyramidical obelisks were built on ley lines, the old tracks. Therefore the economic development plan was simple.

"Ley lines attract people, they allow pilgrims to walk with the energy from one place to another, so let us build pyramids on the leys because they have good energies too. People get twice the value."

"Sound advice," said another ancient developer. "Why don't we build temples and erect obelisks with the magic roofs?"

"And academies...and market places...and inns for travelers to stay," cried another with growing excitement.

Some might think this is fictional stuff but far from it. New York City's Fifth Avenue and St. Patrick's Cathedral were built on leys, in Philadelphia Broad and Market Streets both run on major leys and in Washington DC the entire city grid, including the Capitol Building and the National Mall is based on leys.

So let us track the ley energies in America.

Whether they be pyramids, obelisks, leys or geospirals they all radiate energies which appeal to the human consciousness. The energies also heal and are excellent places for the human body to rest upon, recuperate from an illness or simply relax and enjoy. While ley lines are rare, geospirals are plentiful and spring up (that's a terrible pun) in the most unexpected places, not just in New Mexico and Egypt, but all over the world. You may have one in your garden, the plot of land next door or the park down the street. All one needs to do is get some dowsing tools and go find them.

After we had written HOLY DIRT, SACRED EARTH, A Dowser's Journey in New Mexico we started to find energy spirals in many other places.

Like the cathedral in Santa Fe where there is a geospiral in the Chapel of the Blessed Sacrament, we found older churches in other states were built on or near geospirals. The Sacred Heart Catholic Church in Mount Holly, New Jersey like the cathedral in Santa Fe has a geospiral in its Chapel of the Blessed Sacrament. People who come for mass during the weekdays find it always relaxing and indeed rejuvenating.

It is not just the old Catholic churches that are built on or near geo-spirals. On the road south from Mount Holly to Juliustown, the traveler will find the Quaker House perched on a plateau downhill from the many graves on Arney's Mount. The plateau also serves as a parking lot and it accommodates no less than five geospirals that manifest an area of influence well into the Quaker House and beyond.

Our new research started in Northern New York where there are many leys and their accompanying geospirals.

# THE ROCHESTER-BIRD ISLAND LEY — 820 MILES

Cosmic energy prevails in Rochester, a city on the southern shores of Lake Ontario where it flanks the Genesee River. Founded as a village in 1817 the energies prevalent in the community attracted numerous bands of explorers, inventors, artists, designers, writers, businessmen and others.

Eastman Kodak, Bausch & Lomb, Xerox, the Gannett Company and Western Union all trace their roots to Rochester.

The world's first digital camera was invented in Rochester in December 1975 by Kodak Eastman engineer Steven Sasson. The eight pound camera recorded 0.01 megapixel black and white photos to a cassette tape. The first photograph took 23 seconds to create. Experts say every year digital cameras around the world take one trillion pictures — all stemming from the creative atmosphere in Rochester. One must not forget it was Kodak in Rochester that invented the Brownie in February 1900. Over 100 models were produced and millions sold over the next 70 years to happy photo-snappers world wide.

What attracted great inventive minds to this northern community? Well, some say it's the earth energies. For a start Rochester is inundated with geospirals radiating positive Yin energy which enhances creativity with large areas of influence. For instance at the Kodak Park there is a small vortex of geospirals — an alpha with 49 rings and at least nine others mostly minors, but all contributing to an area of influence of at least half a mile. There's also a leyline, an old track that runs through the city.

If the ley seeker walks along the Genesee River bank towards the U.S. Coastguard Station there is an invisible triple-haired leyline that comes across Lake Ontario and heads south. It crosses the US Post Office in the Central Business District, flanks the 1st Universalist Church, Washington Square Park and passes through the Geva Theater Center.

Destination? It sweeps through the wild hills, forests and streams of western Pennsylvania to a great place of learning that started in 1855 as the Farmers' High School of Pennsylvania. Today it is State College, Pennsylvania State University with almost 9,000 academics and over 98,000 students.

The ley sweeps through, where else? The Meridian on College Avenue, where many students live.

Again, there are many geospirals impregnating the college area with positive, creative energy and the farmers back in 1855 must have known the energy when they selected the site for their school.

The Rochester ley sweeps south and in Charlottesville Virginia passes through Purley Middle School and flanks the Mary Williams Community Center inside the Jefferson School City Center. It misses the Lewis & Clark and Sacagawea Statue at the West Main Street and Ridge Street by a few feet. The monument commemorates the 1803-1806 journey of the Lewis and Clark Expedition. The statue was sculpted by Charles Keck, a prominent sculptor of his day. Commissioned by Paul Goodloe McIntire and given to the citizens of Charlottesville in 1919.

There's a leyline and Native Indian connection here. The statue is located in a prominent historic and geographic position in Charlottesville that predates the settlement of the town. Main Street was once called Three Notch'd Road, constructed in the 1730's by improving an old Monacan Indian trail to allow travel between Richmond and the Shenandoah Valley.

During the Civil War, Midway Hospital was located just to the east of the statue, on the grounds of what is now Midway Manor Apartments. The figures of Lewis, Clark and Sacajewea face west, and are considered historically accurate with lovely proportions and beautiful details. To appreciate the statue fully, the visitor should look carefully at the base of the statue, where the written descriptions are supplemented by carvings which represent significant aspects of their journey.

The Rochester Ley's last point before it heads off into the Atlantic is the southern tip of Bird Island State Reserve, a much loved sand dunes and white beaches region saved from housing developers and now protected for all time.

Towards the end of September countless thousands of northern New Yorkers pack their bags and travel south to escape the hazards of winter and enjoy the sunshine of Florida, the Carolinas and Louisiana. It's the "great snow-bird migration" as one punster described it.

Many of the Rochester folk are no different, in fact ask a few and they will say they are heading for the golden sands and golf courses at Myrtle Beach in South Carolina. Bird Island with its powerful ley and geospirals is a short hop to the Myrtle Beach vacation mecca. Which raises the question do people subconsciously follow ley lines?

FOR DOWSERS: Coordinates.
Rochester / Genesee River: 43°15′23.80″ N 77°36′08.60″ W
State College PA. The Meridian: 40°48′03.23″ N 77°51′51.04″ W
Charlottesville, VA. Lewis & Clarke: 38°01′49.48″ N 78°29′07.03″ W
Bird Island Preserve, North Carolina: 33°51′01.93″ N 78°32′36.29″ W

# CAPE VINCENT AND THE FRENCH CONNECTION

Every Saturday after the Fourth of July thousands of people flock to the tiny historic village of Cape Vincent which stands where the waters of Lake Ontario flow into the St. Lawrence River and they create fabulous vistas among its famous Thousand Islands.

They come to see, photograph and cheer the French Emperor Napoleon Bonaparte resplendent in uniform and sitting on a white charger heading a parade of dazzling floats, all the while munching the delights of pâtisseries françaises. It is all part of the French Festival which has taken place one weekend every year for almost half a century.

Napoleon Bonaparte? The fellow whose Grande Armée occupied Egypt, carted off ancient obelisks and is alleged to have encountered a spirit while visiting the Great Pyramid at Giza?

"Oui, monsieur. The very same. You understand, here it is an imitation."

"Of course! But why?"

"To celebrate the fact he did not come, monsieur. Can you imagine? Beaucoup de problèmes?"

Some Cape people say it is all a myth. Others say it could have happened. So if the dowser makes tracks along Broadway and turns right on Real Street at number 157 you will be standing outside the Cape Vincent

Community Library flanking the great St. Lawrence River. You will also be standing on a ley and a bunch of geospirals.

It was here, just over two hundred years ago that a Frenchman Compte Pierre François Réal, a Parisian lawyer and the prefect of police in Napoleon Bonaparte's regime settled in the community. Immediately he started building a unique house that appeared very strange because it resembled an inverted cup on a saucer and became known as "The Cup and Saucer House." The basement contained a large wine cellar and above on the main floor which was the saucer, were the ordinary living rooms surrounded by a wide and expansive veranda overlooking the water. The main floor in today's lingo would be "open area" because the only walls were built-in screens resting on casters that could be moved to make small rooms or one large room.

The house was decorated with oil paintings, mostly of the Emperor and his marshals. Fireplaces and mantels were intricately carved in European style while silver and gold candlesticks and candelabra illuminated every area, including a library and music area which contained a Stradivarius violin.

Upstairs in the domed section were two rooms. One was a laboratory and the other was a study which contained relics and souvenirs from Napoleon's personal collection brought over to America by Compte Pierre Francois Réal.

There was only one thing missing: The Emperor.

It was October 1815 and Napoleon had lost the Battle of Waterloo and the British Government had placed him in exile on the island of Saint Helena, a volcanic and tropical rock measuring ten by five miles in the Southern Atlantic from where escape was considered impossible. It is over one thousand miles and more from anywhere.

But to the French minds gathered in far off Cape Vincent in upstate New York impossible was not an option. The special house built by Compte Réal was intended as a home for his master, the Emperor of France and Réal and his allies plotted for his escape.

The plotters who met at the Cape included Marquis Emmanuel de Grouchy, General Jean Francois Rolland, Camille Arnaud, Paul

Charboneau and the young brothers Louis and Hyacinthe Peugnet who had been second lieutenants in Napoleon's Imperial Army. The odd man out of this group was a character named Professor Pigeon who was listed as secretary to Compte Réal but was also an accomplished astronomer. Why did the Frenchman need a man accomplished in the planets and stars when in reality he needed someone knowledgeable in Earth energy? Like leys and geospirals.

Today, the Cape Vincent Community Library now stands on the site of Compte Réal's Teacup and Saucer House. It was built not only on a triple-haired ley line but on a blind spring that produces a number of geospirals. The energy radiating from these two elements can be felt even if you just stand in the street or sit yourself down for a while on the chairs at the back of the library. The Area of Influence is substantial. Summer visitors staying at the house next door said: "Energy? The place is full of good, positive energy. Very relaxing. Why do you ask?" Betty Lou took time out to explain.

Back to Réal's group. The conspirators met regularly and in secret at Cape Vincent to discuss news from Europe and St. Helena and shared views on the possibility of rescuing their beloved Emperor. Their hopes were dashed in the summer of 1821 when news arrived that Napoleon Bonaparte had died from stomach cancer on May 5th. Aged 51 he had been imprisoned on the island for five years . In 1840 his body was returned to Paris where it was interred in the Dóme des Invalides in a tomb by the altar. Ironically, Compte Real may have wanted Napoleon to live on a ley in Cape Vincent, but his tomb at the majestic Dóme des Invalides is also on a ley not mentioned in this study.

When a better political climate occurred in France, most of Réal's group, including Réal returned to their native land, except the Peugnet brothers, they took over the homes of the departed. Their younger brother Theophilius who joined them at Cape Vincent, moved into the Cup and Saucer House and lived there until it was destroyed by fire on October 14, 1867.

All the Peugnets, except Louis are buried in the St. Vincent de Paul cemetery in Cape Vincent. Their spirit lives on because in 2009 the Great,

Great Grand Niece of Louise Peugnet visited the cemetery and renovated one of the stained glass windows in the adjoining St. Vincent de Paul Church. Her name: Patrice Cecile Peugnet.

Meanwhile back in time the energies prevalent in Cape Vincent and Réal's core group attracted many veterans of Napoleon's Grand Armée to migrate and settle in the region. The names of the original settlers are still carried by their many descendants — Gosier, Docteur, Dezengremel, Mussot, Chavoustie, Favrey, Merchant, Majo and more.

The visitor can view the many grave markers at the Pioneer Cemetery between Cape Vincent and Rosiere. Bourcey, Wiley, Branche, Margrey, Zimmerman, Reff, Rehm, Mason, Kimmis, the list goes on indicating the strong northern European origin of the Cape Vincent-Rosiere pioneers. Their remains are also clad in strong Earth energies.

A stone's throw away along Dezengremel Road is a grassy plateau with an official State sign which reads: *French Catholic Church built here 1832 by early settlers. Heroes of Napoleon's Army and French refugees worshiped here.*

Nearby is a white altar with a cross.

Regardless of what religion or spiritual background you hold, when you sit on the monument's steps you will feel the relaxing and healing energies radiating from a blind spring that is producing at least nineteen geospirals, one of them a maximum 49-ring phenomenon. We dowsed the Area of Influence of this small vortex. It spans one half mile in any direction from the monument and it appropriately includes the resting place of the pioneers.

The energy is there for all who stop by at the white memorial. When Satchmo, one of our two Chihuahuas hurt a hind leg Betty Lou and I would often on a summer's evening take the dogs and sit with them for 20 minute healing sessions at the Rosiere vortex.

Some might consider it a great pity the original pioneers' church was replaced by another more modern church in the heart of the village of Rosiere. Little remains of the original church but if you are skilled in elementary dowsing you can still find the heads of stone posts indicating the foundations.

One wonders who was the dowser or sensitive who declared back in the 1830s "the energy here is a good place to build our church." On a quiet summer's evening as the bats fly high over the nearby barns and an owl murmurs a hoot, you may well hear distant voices — echoes of the past from another dimension. Incidentally, after sitting in the energy for fifteen perhaps twenty minutes, you may feel so relaxed you may notice a distinct reluctance to get up and leave. It happens. That's the geospirals phenomenon with a distinctly French and Napoleonic touch. Enjoy.

FOR DOWSERS:
Rosiere Monument, NY Coordinates 44°06′36.95" N 76°15′16.22" W

# TEACUP AND SAUCER LEY

The ley comes across the St. Lawrence River from Canada, passes through where the old Teacup and Saucer House used to be, now the Cape Vincent Library, and then heads south to Henderson Harbor. There is a strong suggestion that this ley continues to Syracuse and passes through the Cathedral of the Immaculate Conception on Columbus Circle. Before it reaches the Circle however it passes through several churches on Montgomery Street. This ley needs dowsing south in the United States and north in Canda.

FOR DOWSERS
CV Community Library: Teacup & Saucer site 44°07′39.71"
N 76°20′22.78" W
Henderson Harbor Boat Ramp: 43°50′55.45" N 76°12′24.29" W
Columbus Circle, Syracuse 43°02′48.65" N 76°08′58.13" W

# WATERTOWN NY — A SLEEPING SHANGRI-LA

"Where more than a couple of ley lines gather and geospirals fill the air with vibrant, attractive energies, people feel the urge to live, create and enjoy the aura." We wrote this in our first energy book which focused on the vast collection of writers, photographers, artists, and egocentrics that gathered in northern New Mexico over the years.

Watertown, nestling along the Black River in the upper reaches of Northern New York State, possesses similar cosmic energies that attract creative people with great ideas and plans.

The region was the original homeland of the Iroquois in upstate New York between the Adirondack Mountains, the St. Lawrence, Lake Ontario and Niagara Falls. Watertown and its immediate environs served as a traditional summer camping and hunting area for the tribes. It is highly likely they knew and enjoyed the Earth energies until the early 1800s when they yielded to land speculators and moved away. Tribes such as the Onondaga, Mohawk and Oneida however stayed and are still active today.

The Earth energies in Watertown made it a key industrial center in the 19th century. The railways enabled New York City residents to escape the humidity of summer and bathe in the attractive cool air and waters of the North Country. Frederick Gilbert Bourne, director and president of the Singer Sewing Machine Company built Singer Castle, George C. Boldt started to build Boldt Castle (which is currently being completed), Irving Berlin purchased a cottage overlooking the St. Lawrence and called it "Always" after his 1925 hit.

The Black River that originates in the foothills of the Adirondacks and sweeps through to Lake Ontario, gave the town its name. Its water power helped spawn one of the early industrial centers. Paper and lumber mills were major industries of the 19th century which in turn attracted railroads along with scores of regional dairy farms, cider mills, cheese factories and a brisk tourist industry for nearby communities — Sackets Harbor, Cape Vincent, Clayton and Alexandria Bay.

Among the many notable people who were either born or lived in Watertown were John Calhoun, founding publisher of the Chicago

Democrat, John Foster Dulles, US Secretary of State and his brother Allen Dulles, Director of the Central Intelligence Agency and Samuel Beardsley, Roswell Flower and Moses Field — all US Congressmen. The list includes singer John Gary, movie actor Viggo Mortensen of "Lord of the Rings", artist Robert Guinan who became famous in Europe, actor Richard Grieco who played Detective Dennis Booker on "21 Jump Street" and its sequel "Booker." Producer, screenwriter, camera operator Mark Neveldine who directed "Ghost Rider: Spirit of Vengeance" plus some 30 other titles came from here.

Great ideas started in Watertown: While working in the town Frank Winfield Woolworth had the idea of a five and dime store which became Woolworth worldwide. 1951 saw the creation of Little Trees air conditioners now owned and manufactured in the town by Car-Freshner Corporation.

The Great Depression hit Watertown in the late 1920s and early 1930s. The annual influx of New York City visitors dwindled not only because of the economy but the advent of portable air conditioners. The railways gradually cut back and almost disappeared.

In 1904 the military started coming to nearby Pine Camp and throughout the ensuing years with steady growth assisted in maintaining the region's economy.

The land around Watertown once a mecca for milk farms and cheese factories is now given to small farms and hay production. Today, the heavy industry that once flanked the Black River has mostly disappeared and the scene is now dominated by kayakers from across the country and indeed overseas who come to challenge the river's white waters.

Understanding the potential of Earth energy one would have thought Watertown NY would possess a more vibrant, bouncing and innovative economy. The energy in the downtown area comes from a series of leys that gather and cross in the once elegant and attractive Public Square.

Watertown NY is a hotbed of Earth energies as we shall see.

The bi-level arcade, the renovated Woolworth building, the impressive stone church, images of a prosperous bygone era are still there on the Square. The magnificent railway station with its awesome Grecian columns and marble floors is long gone erased by an erroneous post-world war II urban renewal plan that captured nothing of the town's old glory.

Memories aside, if one ignores the endless streams of non-stop traffic and perhaps sits on one of the benches that adorn the Square's center island, the energy is evident. You may wander inside the offices of the North Country Arts Council where artists of every brush, photographers and writers gather, chat and display their works and then hang around, you will feel it. Of course the Arts Council has it home here. It is natural and so it organizes events under the banner "Arts on the Square."

It is little wonder because in addition to the cris-cross of ley energies there is a massive blind spring under the town producing at least 44 geospirals with one or more at 49 rings. It is very difficult to physically count a large geospiral in a commercial area so one has to resort to a pendulum count.

For those who are aware of Earth energies Watertown is a natural attraction for creative arts, innovation, education, natural healing and simply relaxing in bistros or walking tree-lined boulevards — all the benefits that come from leys and geospirals.

Hanging out is one of the encouraging powers of geospirals, but there is more. One of three ley lines runs through the Arts Center and another two run through the Public Square, in fact anywhere one stands in the area, one can sense the relaxing and healing energy of the leys and the geospirals.

Let us take a look.

# THE INDIAN RIVER-WATERTOWN- POINT PENINSULA LEY

Indian River village is a tiny community on NY Route 812 made fascinating by the fact its General Store is surprisingly but happily installed in an old church. The ley running east-west can be found between the store and the Erie Canal Road. Almost on a direct west run, it passes through downtown Carthage crossing North Main near Bridge Street then heads for the north sidewalk at Watertown's Public Square. It comes close to Dexter before heading for Point Peninsula and the famous Little White Church and the Shangri-la community before heading off into Lake Ontario. Point Peninsula is a hotbed for geospirals. We counted 19 with at least one manifesting 49 rings.

One Rochester resident sitting on the beach outside the Shangri-la Resort said: "This is my 35th summer here. No place like it for relaxing and feeling good. Pull up a chair and stay awhile."

We did. The restaurant is famous for its fish and chips.

FOR DOWSERS: Coordinates:
Indian River Village, NY 43°58'26.78" N 75°22'13.89" W.
Carthage: N. Main near Bridge St., 43°58'27.00" N 75°36'55.22" W
Watertown Sq. N sidewalk: 43°58'29.40" N 75°54'34.01" W
Little White Church, Point Peninsula NY 44°00'23.28" N 76°13'05.72" W

Note: There are indications of another ley near the South Shore/Pine Woods intersection on Point Peninsula.

# THE BOLDT CASTLE-WATERTOWN-CHITTENANGO LEY

On many summer weekends a visitor is guaranteed to witness a wedding taking place on an island in the middle of the St. Lawrence River and Seaway. If you stand or sit there and watch for a while you will notice how relaxed and easy you feel. Not a care in the world. Some may think it is the wedding or the old world castle with its strange rock-built tower called the Dovecote that stands majestically behind the happy couple. Some may think it is the power of romance that surrounds Boldt Castle, the majestic home that New York hotelier George Boldt started to build for his love Louise. But all was immediately abandoned when his wife died.

Earth energy is subtle and chances are the relaxation and well-being that you feel is because a tripled-haired ley runs through the bridal path leading up to the Dovecote and actually enters the tower by the doorway. Mr. Boldt created a circle of tiles inside the building and the ley runs right through the center. If you have never heard of a dovecote it is a structure for housing pigeons. Inside the massive rock tower the focal point of a set of tiles is precisely set on the center of the ley.

It now raises the question did Mr. Boldt know of the ley or was the Dovecote built where it stands by sheer intuition. We shall probably never know. One thing more. The island is laced with geospirals continually bathing the area in relaxing and inspiring energy for couples launching their married life or for people just to hang out there.

Dowsers can find this ley a short distance north of Rockport on the Waterfront Trail. The town has been the scene of boat building on the St. Lawrence for over 200 years and today is the home of Rockport Boat Line and Ed Huck Marine. The energy line runs almost due south across the St. Lawrence River.

It crosses Heart Island the home of Boldt Castle and on the mainland heads for the north-east end of the River Hospital in Alexandria Bay. From there it heads to Watertown.

The line crosses the Public Square a few paces east of the Woolworth Building then in a well-calculated move passes through the YMCA and then the Roswell P. Flower Memorial Library both on Washington Street.

It is interesting in that four very attractive buildings designed to benefit people are all built on a leyline which also manifests geospiral energies — Boldt Castle, River Hospital, the YMCA and a very large Memorial Library.

The ley continues almost directly due south crossing the Samaritan Summit Village which provides multiple levels of support for the local senior population, including an entirely new level of care for the community — assisted living. Leaving Watertown the ley is next picked up east of Cleveland and then crosses Oneida Lake to a village east of Syracuse called Chittenango.

Chittenango? Be there the first week of June and you'll think you are in the famous Land of Oz because there is the Yellowbrick Road and everyone is attired just like the great characters in the famous movie which starred Judy Garland, Frank Morgan, Ray Bolger, Jack Haley and Margaret Mitchell who played the Wicked Witch.

Why? The man who wrote the book in 1934 *The Wonderful Wizard of Oz*, consequently filmed as "The Wizard of Oz" in 1939

was L. Frank Baum born in Chittenango on May 15<sup>th</sup> 1856.

The village holds an annual festival for three days called Oz-Stravaganza! honoring Baum's life and literary works.

Appropriately the ley is just off Highway 5 or Genesee Street. It crosses the rear of the building where many books are found, the Sullivan Free Library. A stone's throw along Genesee Street is the All Things Oz Museum.

FOR DOWSERS: Coordinates:
Rockport, CA a short distance north on Waterfront Trail.
44° 23′14.09" N 75° 55′45.72" W.
Boldt Castle NY Dovecote, 44°20′41.56" N 75°55′34.01" W
Watertown NY Public Square: On sidewalk outside Woolworth
43° 58′29.29" N 75° 54′38.03" W
Chittenango NY: Sullivan Free Library. 43°02′38.67" N 75°51′57.06" W

# THE KINGSTON-WATERTOWN-LOWVILLE LEY

We first discovered this ley by sheer accident and it triggered the start of this book. During the summer months when we are in upstate New York, Betty Lou and I like to walk with the Chihuahuas along the old railway right of way between Watertown and Cape Vincent. It is an invigorating walk as we discovered.

You may recall our mentioning a meadow to which Betty Lou was drawn and we discovered a whole nest of geospirals that had once served as a Native Indian summer camp. We pointed out it flanks the old railway right of way.

Although the passenger trains stopped plying the rails in the spring of 1936 and the steel tracks were removed during World War II, there are still remnants. The stone pillars of the bridge at Chaumont still stand proudly above the river bed and occasionally a wooden tie (sleeper if you are English) that supported the rails will raise its head through the grasses that have grown along the track to cry: "We are still here, folks!"

If on a quiet summer's evening a walker pauses to take in the aroma of the countryside and its history, one may still hear the sounds of the old steam locomotives trundling along and perhaps the happy voices of tourists heading for the Cape. This is what prompted the ghostly Sunset Train that became an important structure in my novel *For the Love of Rose: A Journey in Three Worlds.*

One August morning when the sun was just starting a climb through a scattering of pink clouds into a blue sky, the grass was still wet with overnight dew, we stopped on the old railway right-of-way.

"There's a voice telling me I should dowse for a leyline," I said to Betty Lou. Thinking back it must have been Bernard before he made his presence clear.

A rod went into the search position and started swinging round and round. I walked back into Betty Lou's meadow, the rod swung back to where she was standing.

"The ley is right there. On the old railway track," I exclaimed attempting not to be excited. With one rod in the Search position we followed it along the old railway line.

. "The railway engineers when they planned this section of the Watertown-Cape Vincent track back in 1840s, they built it on a ley line!"

It was a discovery that would take us on various dowsing expeditions. before I learned to map dowse on Google Earth.

Google Earth showed that the railway track was only straight at a point south of Rosiere Station through the villages of Three Mile Bay and Chaumont to a point near Limerick, a total distance of about 13 miles.

The ley then heads through Brownville, passing through the historic stone mansion of Major General Jacob Brown who introduced organized recruiting in the U.S. Army. No desk soldier, he became a war hero in the armed and totally useless conflict between the United States and the British Empire known as the War of 1812.

The ley sweeps on into Watertown's Public Square and passes through the Jefferson County Offices including the NY State Supreme Court Law

Library before heading along the north side of the Square, clipping the impressive stone First Baptist Church with its tower at the east end. The ley then generally parallels State Street, State Route 12 to Lowville where it drops by the offices of the Journal and Republican newspaper which has been serving the community since 1860. The ley then crosses a field north of the Walmart Super Store where it crosses another ley before heading off into the Black River Wild Forest.

# THE CANADIAN CONNECTION

On the other end of this ley, the energy line leaves Rosiere and heads for the St. Lawrence River, crossing Route 12E at the entrance to Willow Shores RV community in Cape Vincent. On Canada's Wolfe Island it crosses 9th Line Road at Memory Lane.

East of Marysville on Route 96 is the working boatyards of MetalCraft Marine Inc. This international firm specializes in custom boat building, conducts research and is a marine training center. The crew create all sorts of water vessels including patrol boats, fireboats, workboats and barges plus handling used boats that are spread across their lot.

Well, the international ley crosses MetalCraft's property. When dowsers are out conducting searches and surveys, occasionally people will come up and ask what we're doing, then walk away shaking their heads. But today was different. A bearded man looked out of a pickup truck and enquired what was happening.

"There's an earth energy line coming from New York State across the St. Lawrence," I said. "We're tracking the line. It's heading for Kingston."

In the conversation that lasted for at least ten minutes, the bearded man who said his name was Tom Wroe, showed a lot of interest when we told him his yard contained several geospirals.

"Your operation must have a lot of good creative energy," I said.

He smiled and nodded. "The water is great. You can get some good pictures at the back of the lot," he said and drove away.

During our stay in the boatyard we found three geospirals with the alpha putting out 35 rings.

Another fellow Kevin McKenna who had been standing nearby said: "It's a great place to work at. It always feels comfortable. The building used to make Kraft cheese, now it's a creative center for boat design.

"Who is Tom Wroe?"

"Oh, he's the boss. President of MetalCraft."

From MetalCraft's property on Wolfe Island you can see downtown Kingston which is a 20-minute free ferryboat ride from Marysville.

Kingston is a city that is a pure dowser's delight. There are a number of powerful leys plus a flotilla of geospirals radiating healthy and relaxing Yin energy. It's little wonder that people have guarded the place since time immemorial because visitors not only soak up history but swamp the body and mind with Earth energy.

The Indian ancestors named the place Cataraqui an Iroquois word that means "the place where one hides" or "place of retreat" or "where the rivers and lake meet". It all depends on whom you encounter. One thing is for sure, the city's origin dates back into the mists of time and it's a great place to hang out and enjoy the energies.

There's archaeological evidence hinting that Native ancestors lived in the Kingston area about 3,000 to 9,000 years ago and early Iroquois were here somewhere between 500 to 1,000 years ago. Everybody who was anybody, hung their hats here. The Hurons, the Mississaugas, the French, the British, the fur trappers and traders. It was also a receiving center for Loyalist refugees who fled north because of the American Revolutionary War.

Cataraqui's name was changed to "the King's Town" in 1787 in honor of Britain's King George III. The name was shortened to "Kingston" in 1788. If you enjoy seeing and photographing buildings of any sort, Kingston is also known as the "Limestone City" because of the many heritage buildings constructed using local limestone.

Kingston became so attractive that it became for a short period the capital of a united Canada. The Canadian Locomotive Company was at one time the largest locomotive works in the British Empire. In

Confederation Park you will find Locomotive 1095 built for the Canadian Pacific Railway. The old engine stands close to the harbor where the Watertown ley comes in from Wolfe Island. This ley can be dowsed at the harbor on the Rideau Trail close to Johnson Street.

The ley heads north-west across Ontario Street and King Street East and passes through another great bookshop owned by the Diocese of Ontario. If you stand by the doorway, you are right on the ley. In the next block it crosses through the Kingston-Frontenac Public Library. There's something about bookshops, libraries and ley lines.

The ley is next recorded at Sydenham Street where it intersects with Brock Street. This is just one block away from the Sydenham-Princess Street intersection where archaeologists have designated the area as the place where the Iroquois ancestors first set up their community almost a thousand years ago. There's something about leys and Native Ancestors too.

FOR DOWSERS: Coordinates north to south.
Diocese of Ontario Bookshop, Kingston 44°13′45.17″ N 76°29′02.20″ W
Rideau Trail (Harbor) Kingston CA. 44°13′39.83″ N 76°28′51.96″ W
Wolfe Island, East of Marysville (MetalCraft) 44°11′55.50″ N 76°25′07.41″ W
Rosiere, NY Rte 4 (100 yds E of old railway) 44°07′14.97″ N 76°14′33.12″ W
Watertown Square, Baptist Church. 43°58′28.11″ N 75°54′28.77″ W
Lowville, NY Journal & Republican. 43°47′09.56″ N 75°29′30.76″ W

# A STRANGE FINDING IN KINGSTON.

Whenever dowsing for a specific event — in this case the Lowville-Watertown-Kingston Ley, there is always something else that just simply crops up and says: Surprise!

Leys around the world are dotted with churches, temples and other holy places and include schools, colleges, libraries, churches and places for arts and fitness.

So we wondered why the Lowville-Watertown-Kingston ley narrowly misses by a physical stone's throw a spiritual and beautiful building created out of limestone, complete with majestic Grecian columns. It is the St. George's Anglican Cathedral standing on the corner of Johnson and King Street East in Kingston.

Curious, Betty Lou and I decided to walk across and see. First of all we found a large geospiral gushing with energy just outside the Cathedral, and then we stumbled on a ley line running parallel to the Grecian columns and crossing the main entrance to the Cathedral. Anyone entering the main doors has to cross over this ley line.

Yes, this ley crosses the Lowville-Watertown-Kingston ley and runs on a nor-nor-east course along King Street East. At Brock the street suddenly turns to an almost northern course, but the ley continues crossing the fronts of several shops until it comes to a tavern called Sir John's Pub and thereby hangs another story.

Who was Sir John?

A young man born in Scotland in the 19th century and took up a life-long residence in Kingston was Sir John Alexander Macdonald. An ambitious young man, he became a Canadian politician and Father of Confederation and thus the first Prime Minister of Canada. A political career which spanned almost half a century, his reign was filled with great events and upheavals. In 1873 Sir John was voted out of office during the famous Pacific Scandal in which his political party took bribes from businessmen seeking the contract to build the Pacific Railway.

Memorials to "Sir John A" as he is known in Kingston are scattered across the Canadian Commonwealth he helped to build. At 343 King Street East the visitor will find Sir John's Pub which occupies the building used by Sir John as his law office from 1849 to 1860.

As we dowsed the ley on this street I casually snapped a photo of Sir John's Pub for our records. As an old professional news photographer I detest the word "snapped" however this is exactly what happened. Returning to base we discovered the picture shows some strange psychic activity. It is included in our album.

The ley goes through other buildings and crosses Princess Street before heading off across the Cataraqui River. For dowsers this ley is worth further tracking.

The energies in Kingston have given rise to a lot of famous people: singer, song writer and photographer Bryan Adams, hockey player Doug Kilmour won the Stanley Cup with the Calgary Flames, Don Cherry, born February 5, 1934 a long time Canadian commentator for CBC Television and Hockey Night in Canada, and Polly Shannon who at this date has been in 64 American and Canadian TV and cinema movies. Polly played Margaret Trudeau in a tv movie on the life of Pierre Elliott Trudeau, prime minister of Canada for almost 16 years.

# A PYRAMID IN CANADA?

Paranormal and UFO sightings are common in eastern Canada, but when a young woman based in Kingston spots a UFO shaped as a pyramid, it draws our attention.

It was early May 1972 when Vicki Cameron with the Royal Canadian Signal Corps, 709 Communications Squadron was stationed in Kingston on a training course.

One evening about dusk Vicki and 13 other communications specialists were returning from exercises. In two vehicles they were driving on the back roads near some little town about 30 miles north of Kingston.

We all saw it, she said. It was like a flying building coming towards them. She gave the command to stop and everyone jumped out and stared. The object in the sky was shaped like a pyramid — the size of a 747 jet aircraft. There were no wings, no fuselage, and the group could not figure out how it was suspended in the sky.

In her book "Don't tell anyone but...UFO EXPERIENCES IN CANADA" she says: "It scared the hell out of us."

Although the group was armed from the exercise, no one fired at the object. The pyramid came within half a kilometer of the service group, hovered, then made a sharp right turn. In the turn it straightened up, so it was vertical. After a few moments it took off at an estimated 600 miles an hour. The whole episode lasted three or four minutes and of course, the group made a report, signed it and gave it to their sergeant. The report was passed to higher echelons — and disappeared.

# DR. TRUDEAU: THE ENERGY CALLED

By the time the 18th century finished, officials estimate that tuberculosis or consumption as it was originally named, had killed one in seven of all people who ever lived on Planet Earth. By the end of the 19th century TB was still a deadly disease, in fact up until World War II no one ever took the disease lightly. In England during the war I lost my Aunt Eydie Daniels and an infant niece.

It was during those 1940 war years that Streptomycin was developed and showed a promising glimmer of hope for patients but it was not to be. It did however show the way. Antibiotics were developed in the 1950s and included para-amino salicylic acid, isoniazid, pyrazinamide, cycloserine, and kanamycin.

TB victims suffered from physically debilitating hacking, bloody coughs, prolonged pain in the lungs and the seemingly ever-lasting fatigue.

In the 19th century doctors were searching frantically for places that possessed qualities conducive to healing tuberculosis. Fresh mountain air was one.

Travelers to the mountains, streams and waterfalls of the Adirondacks in upstate New York will likely recall the vast forests of red spruce, white pine, sugar maple and American beech. They monopolize nearly every corner of the great wilderness park. If one stands and admires the incredible and majestic views one cannot fail to feel the freshness of the air, the all invigorating oxygen bathing one's lungs and body.

Perched high in these mountains is Saranac Lake which in modern times basks in historic memories.

If you had come this way in the 1880s and for the next sixty or so years, you would have witnessed strange and eerie sights. Clusters of people, sitting on wide and open verandas, balconies and patios, all wrapped up in furs and heavy coats and all breathing the clean and very cold mountain airs — even with heavy snow cloaking everything.

They were victims of an ancient and often fatal disease, tuberculosis, and this was the age of the Sanatorium.

Enter Edward Livingston Trudeau, a young doctor from New York City who had already had a severe encounter with TB. He nursed his older brother for three months before death claimed him. In marriage the Trudeaus lost three of their four children to tuberculosis.

It was when Dr. Trudeau now with a practice on Long Island, contracted TB himself that colleagues suggested a change of air. One suggested Northern New York. Desperate, he headed north.

In the Adirondack Mountains he spent as much time as possible in the open air and subsequently regained his health. It was as if he had discovered a panacea. In 1876 he moved his family to Saranac Lake and established a medical practice among the sportsmen, guides and lumber camps of the region.

In 1882, Dr. Trudeau read about Prussian Dr. Hermann Brehmer's success treating tuberculosis with the "rest cure" in cold, clear mountain air. Through this concept Trudeau founded the Adirondack Cottage Sanitarium, with the support of several of the wealthy businessmen. The remedy for tuberculosis was fresh air and nutritious foods.

Fire destroyed his small laboratory in 1884 so the doctor organized the Saranac Laboratory for the Study of Tuberculosis with a gift from Elizabeth Milbank Anderson, philanthropist and advocate for public health and women's education. It was the first laboratory in the United States for the study of tuberculosis. Renamed the Trudeau Institute, the laboratory continues today to study infectious diseases.

The Saranac Laboratory also still stands today and serves as a fascinating museum with medical instruments hanging on the walls and patient beds. The staff display movies filmed in the years when the facility was at its prime. Visitors witness artefacts of medical history at 89 Church St # 2, Saranac Lake, NY which was the laboratory and a sort distance away outside the Trudeau Institute building fully preserved is the first cottage that formed part of the historic Sanitarium. It's called Little Red and dates back to 1895. Some of the old houses with large balconies where patients used to sit, wrapped up in furs, scarves, mufflers and gloves and breathing the cold mountain air, still exist on Adirondack Road, although they have long been closed in.

One of Trudeau's early patients was author Robert Louis Stevenson. Among his many patients were celebrities, politicians, authors, businessmen, teachers, scholars and many men and women who were drawn to Saranac because they believed in his work and because the energy was right.

In 2014 when I was writing my novel For the Love of Rose: a journey in three worlds Betty Lou and I visited Saranac Lake to conduct research for use in the book. It was then that we discovered two things: an abundance of geospirals and the existence of a powerful leyline that stretches from Canada down to the Gulf of Mexico. It runs through many of the cottages in the Trudeau Park, passes across the Pine Street bridge before heading for the Trudeau Laboratory Museum on Church Street.

Was Dr. Trudeau a dowser? There are no records to say he was but he must have sensed that Saranac Lake was the right place to build the country's first tuberculosis Sanitarium. If and when you visit, pause for a few minutes and feel the Earth energy manifesting itself. If you feel you need to stay, that's normal. That's one of the powerful attractions of the geospirals and ley energies.

I sense that Dr. Trudeau knew it and stayed there for the rest of his life. He died November 15th 1915 and is buried along with his wife Charlotte in the family plot at St. John's in the Wilderness Episcopal Church in the nearby hamlet of Paul Smiths, New York.

Work was carried on by his son, Francis Trudeau MD. The slow end of the Sanatarium started in 1944 when an effective drug, streptomycin was developed. By the mid-1950s, Sanitarium treatment of tuberculosis was nearly entirely done by drug treatment.

Sixty-three of the hundreds of cure cottages still exist in Saranac Lake and have been placed on the National Register of Historic Places.

On May 12, 2008, the United States Postal Service issued a 76 cent stamp picturing Trudeau, part of the Distinguished Americans series. His descendants include cartoonist Garry Trudeau, a great grandson of the famous doctor.

# THE SARANAC LEY

The surveyed section of this triple-haired ley stretches from a suburb of Montreal, Canada to the Gulf of Mexico, a distance of 1,500 miles and it may even be longer in Canada. This ley is notable for the fact it shares its Earth energies with various educational and health facilities.

At Brossard, a part of Greater Montreal, the ley is found running through L'ecole George P. Vanier, a school set up to commemorate the first francophone governor of Canada.

At Saranac Lake the ley runs through Adirondack Park where many of the Sanitarium cottages were situated, then crosses the Saranac River at the Pine Street bridge. At Church Street the ley goes through Dr. Trudeau's Saranac Laboratory Museum. This whole area is inundated with geospiral energies: One 49 rings plus 11 smaller circles. The area of influence is almost a mile.

At Utica the ley crosses Interstate 90 and the Mohawk River Dam, east of Leland. This city has a tremendous history. All the Mohawk, Onondaga and Oneida tribes surely recognized and used the great energy manifesting itself here, not for the ley but the nest of geospirals, a small vortex that radiates Yin energy throughout the old downtown area and beyond.

Yin is an encouraging energy which is probably one reason, Utica has produced so many ambitious screen and theater people. Top among the long list is Annette Funicello who was under contract to Walt Disney for many years and appeared in a series of "Beach Party" movies.

The ley runs through Bagg Square, once the site of Fort Schuyler, many of the early settlements and the existing historic St. John's Church which dates back to 1821.

It was here among positive earth energies that a young woman named Marianne received her first Holy Communion and Confirmation. A German-born American, a member of the Sisters of St. Francis of Syracuse, NY she spent many years among the lepers on the island of Moloka in Hawaii and was never afflicted by the disease — considered by some to be a miracle. She crossed into Spirit in 1918 at 80 years. In 2005 she was beatified as Saint Marianne Cope, O.S.F.

For dowsers the center of the alpha geospiral is among the trees opposite the main doors and steps of St. John's Church on John Street.

Binghamton: The Saranac ley continues south towards Pennsylvania. It crosses Interstates 85 and 81 and US Route 11 where they meet south-east of Binghamton at Five Mile Point right by the Susquehanna River.

Reading: This Pennsylvania town is another example suggesting the early settlers were either highly intuitive or dowsers or both. In 1748, the town was laid out by Thomas and Richard Penn, the sons of William Penn. The name was chosen after Penn's own county seat, Reading in Berkshire, England. In 1752, Reading became the county seat of Berks county. Fifth Street follows the leyline, in fact on North Fifth the ley is on the east side and gradually moves onto the west side on South Fifth. The coordinates were taken at the Penn Street intersection. One interesting aspect of Fifth Street is the number of schools, churches and libraries flanking the route. Dowsers: Check out the high possibility of geospiral activity.

Aberdeen Proving Grounds, Maryland is also on the Saranac Ley. This is the U.S. Army's oldest active proving ground established in 1917 on the shores of Chesapeake Bay in Hafford County to provide a site for army-materiel testing. Nearby Edgewood Arsenal was also established to provide a site for chemical warfare material development, production and testing. The installations were merged in 1971.

The installation covers more than 72,500 acres, half of which is water or wetlands. Facilities include medical research, chemical, physics, materials and human engineering -laboratories. Aberdeen Proving Ground also is host to National Guard and U.S. Army Reserve operations and training. It employs more than 21,000 military, civilian and contractor employees, making it Hafford County's largest employer. Personnel are responsible for technical achievements in military intelligence, engineering, computer technology and medical research.

The Saranac Ley continues: Moving south we find the energy in such places as the U.S. Naval Academy at Annapolis, Maryland, specifically Bancroft Hall.

The ley can also be found at Roanoke, Virginia and the Mill Mountain Discovery Center which offers opportunities for all ages to explore the natural world through award-winning outreach programs that focus on wildlife, geology, ecology, flora and fauna, and natural history. For 15,000 years this part of the world had strong ties to Native American tribes. Tutelo, Monacan, Iroquois, Cherokee, and Shawnee lived and traded in the area, drawn to the abundant game.

At Tallahassee, Florida we find the ley running through the A & M University Developmental Research School. It is part of FAMU — Florida Agricultural and Mechanical University which has a varied history starting in 1887. The school was originally known as "Lucy Moten" and according to *Notable Black American Women* by Shirelle Phelps "Lucy Ellen Moten's strong influence as an educator of black school teachers changed Washington D.C.'s entire educational system."

A dowser can track the physical end of the Saranac Ley as it continues through the Florida community of Panacea in Wakulla County. Specifically the end on solid ground is on the beach at Alligator Point where the line enters the deep blue waters of the Gulf of Mexico after running almost 1,500 miles.

FOR DOWSERS:
Tracking the Saranac Ley:
Brossard, Canada. L'ecole George P. Vanier 45°27′56.30" N 73°26′54.42" W
Trudeau's Saranac Laboratory Museum 44°19′49.53" N 74°07′45.80" W
Utica NY: Interstate 90 east of Leland 43°01′21.22" N 75°12′29.34" W
Binghamton NY: Five Mile Point by Susquehanna River.
42°05′41.24" N 75°49′41.55" W.
Reading PA: Penn Street intersection. 40°20′07.26" N 75°55′39.93" W
Aberdeen Proving Ground Md. 39°28′37.50" N 76°08′10.48" W

U.S. Naval Academy at Annapolis, Md. specifically Bancroft Hall 38°58′53.78" N 76°28′59.41" W

Roanoke, Va: Mill Mountain Discovery Center 37°14′59.90" N 79°56′05.92" W

At Tallahassee, Florida A & M University Developmental Research School: 30°24′46.22" N 84°17′05.85" W

Panacea Fla. On the beach at Alligator Point 29°53′41.53" N 84°22′49.35" W

Note for dowsers: There may be another ley at the current headquarters of the Trudeau Institute by Lower Saranac Lake.

# AN "INDIAN BURIAL GROUND" THAT IS DIFFICULT TO LEAVE

Somewhere tucked away amid the oaks, beech trees and poison ivy and other greenery that make up the West Amwell Forest the dowsing rods point to an old Native Indian Burial Ground. It's on a rocky, heavily forested shelf at a point east of Lambertville, New Jersey.

How did we find it?

Recently we visited our dowsing friends Dan and Joyce Hofstetter at their home in West Amwell. They were interested in dowsing and suggested we visit and check out the energies in and around their forest home.

The rods indicated a nest of geospiral energies all radiating relaxing and healing Yin energies with the alpha geospiral radiating 28 rings. Such a geospiral is great for living a healthy life, not too strong, not too weak.

It was while we were dowsing Don and Joyce's property that spirits appeared and said the area had been a regular seasonal camping area for Native Indian tribes. They also indicated that the forest area contained a Native Indian Burial Ground which caught most people by surprise.

On Saturday, June 7th 2014 an explorative group convened at the Hofstetter place with a plan to try and find the ancient burial ground via the art of dowsing. The group comprised my partner Betty Lou Kishler, Dan and Joyce Hofstetter, Joanne Pfleiderer, Mark Sterner, and Lori and Lee Hofstetter who live nearby. Their dog Lucky also came along.

Dowsing rods in a search position indicated a north-west direction and for a few yards we walked along the old Rock Road that General George Washington and his men had marched on their way from Lambertville to the battle of Monmouth in 1778.

Dan then led the way along a number of deer tracks and across some clear areas, always in the north-west direction. After almost 30 minutes of hiking through challenging brush, fallen trees and walking through rockfields we came to an area where there were fewer trees but a number of heavy rocks.

Suddenly the search rod spun round. "We have arrived," I announced and everyone started looking around.

The entire area, the size of a baseball infield, was surrounded by rocks that looked like sleeping sentinels and beyond lay some fallen trees almost acting as barriers. Everyone agreed that the energy made this place special. But there was nothing to announce that this was indeed an old Native Indian Burial Ground. However the dowsing rods insisted, so we went along with that.

We knew from our earlier explorations that Native Indians always sought out places that manifested positive Earth energies — in other words geospirals.

"Show me the nearest major geospiral," I asked the search rod. It swung round and stopped just a few feet away. I placed a flag marker at the center and then walked with the rods to count the rings. An impressive thirty-five!

All in all there are at least eight minor geospirals working at this spot. It is little wonder the Lenape Indians used this place to care for the bodies of loved ones in Spirit. The rods indicated the last burial here was 1710.

"Check for ley lines?" said a voice. I did. We found one running right through center of the Indian Burial Ground. The rods showed a triple-haired leyline running north-south.

One of the major attributes of a major geospiral complex or vortex is that visitors experience a distinct reluctance to leave. The force is so beautiful and relaxing it begs the visitor to stay. So Betty Lou and I sat on a rock, she smoked her Indian Peace Pipe and the others practiced with their dowsing rods and pendulums and discussed the phenomenon of being on a place where the earth energy felt sacred. The Native Indians, presumably the Lenape, must have had similar thoughts. A good, sacred place to bury loved ones and a far cry from pyramids.

The trail, if you can call it that, into and out of the burial area is so overgrown that we were surprised to see the appearance of a cross-country cyclist complete with helmet, garb and music plugs. He stopped suddenly.

Everyone asked him where we were and he suggested various trails. I felt he was lost, but then he quickly disappeared down a track we knew was blocked by heavy fallen trees.

It's strange that whenever Betty Lou and I experience a mystical event, a cyclist turns up out of nowhere, makes some comments and disappears. With me it first happened in Cornwall, England, then with Betty Lou when we were at the Kelly's Mine Ghost site in New Mexico, and now in Amwell Forest, New Jersey. Cyclists with messages.

It was during this time at the Indian Burial Ground that I noticed we were being watched by the spirits of the ancestors, perhaps fifty of them standing among the trees. Then I heard a very clear voice in soft English : "Do not disturb this place. Please do not disturb the earth. It is sacred." Thinking back, I think it was from Bernard.

Quickly I mentioned it to the group and everyone agreed, except one — Lori and Lee's pit-bull Lucky. The dog suddenly started digging part of the track, it's claws pulling at the dark rich earth. Lee said it was for eucalyptus roots but some feared it might be something embarrassing. The Lenape were known for shallow burials. Lucky developed such a frenzy that we decided to move out before the hole got any bigger.

Led by Dan the group found its way back and eventually walked along the remains of the ancient Rock Road linking Lambertville to West Amwell.

The Hofstetter property is an ideal area for training both new and experienced dowsers because as I mentioned, it contains a cluster of geo-spirals in a beautiful forest setting. It also contains a geopathic negative energy zone formed by cracks in the rocks deep underground but it is a safe distance from the house. When a dowser finds such a place for practicing dowsing and learning about energies, it should be protected and kept safe.

That is why there are no coordinates for this chapter. Besides it is time to see the big cities.

# TWO LEYS THAT CROSS A CATHEDRAL

Whoever planned St. Patrick's Cathedral in New York City knew exactly what they were doing when it came to Earth energy. It was probably Archbishop John Hughes or renowned architect James Renwick who in the 1850s decided the Cathedral's boundaries would be between Fifth and Madison Avenues and Fiftieth and Fifty-First Streets.

Maybe they felt it was the "right thing to do" or "the place feels good" or perhaps "an angel told us." Perhaps either one or both consulted a dowser. Whatever happened the Cathedral was built on two leys that virtually meet in the shape of a Christian cross. The place is filled with Earth energies from a blind spring manifesting geospirals. It is not as if the leys were "close" or "on the steps," they meet dead center where the Nave meets the Transept. The alpha geospiral's center is between the Crypt and the Lady Chapel. It is a place where the energy is so right. Let us examine the leys.

THE RADIO CITY– CATHEDRAL LEY: This east-west ley is first found on Roosevelt Island at Southpoint Park. The island was once home to the Lenape who called it Minnehanonck. It crosses the East River and moves at a slight southern inclination along 51st Street. It runs through the historic Lotte New York Palace hotel, crosses Madison and runs directly through the Nave at St. George's Cathedral, across Fifth Avenue into the Rockefeller Center and on through Radio City Music Hall across the Avenue of the Americas and heads towards the Hudson River at the end of West 49th and Pier 88 Cruise Ship Terminal.

For Dowsers the coordinates:
Roosevelt Island 40°45′07.01" N 73°57′31.37" W
St. Patrick's Cathedral 40°45′30.64" N 73°58′33.90" W
Radio City Music Hall 40°45′36.04" N 73°58′48.68" W
Hudson / W 49th cruiseship terminal 40°45′57.28" N 73°59′50.95" W

# HARLEM-CATHEDRAL-FULTON FERRY LEY

The north end of this ley is found at the intersection of W 153rd Street and 7th Avenue in Harlem and runs through the New York Housing Authority complex. It then heads south running the full length of Central Park, crossing the Jacqueline Kennedy Onassis Reservoir. It then flows on East Drive between two key points — the so called Cleopatra's Needle and the Metropolitan Museum of Art on the other. Both points are close enough to share the ley's Area of Influence.

The ley crosses 5th Avenue to the East side at the intersection of 59th Street. Nine blocks further south the ley cuts across the middle of St. Patrick's Cathedral, crossing the Radio City — Cathedral Ley as it does so. It then heads through Lower Manhattan and New York University Village, Chinatown, the Financial District and finally the Battery Maritime Building next to the Staten Island Ferry Terminus. The ley goes on to cross the two west-east leys mentioned below.

For Dowsers:
Harlem: W 153rd and 7th Avenue. 40°49′36.15" N 73°56′08.45" W
Needle & MM of Art. East Drive. 40°46′45.23" N 73°57′53.79" W
St. Patrick's Cathedral, Fifth Ave. 40°45′31.68" N 73°58′34.38" W
Battery Maritime next to SI Ferry.40°42′04.07" N 74°00′42.54" W

Note 1: While we were studying this area, we were confused over finding another line, an east-west ley crossing the actual Grand Army Plaza monument in the corner of Central Park at W 59th Street and Fifth Avenue.

Note 2: There is indication of another ley, running north-south found in the vicinity of the Fulton Ferry Terminal near the south end of Brooklyn Bridge.

This is for other dowsers to explore.

# LONG ISLAND AND TWO MASSAPEQUA LEYS

Long Island has two ley lines found in the Massapequa Preserve lands and both cross each other in Hempstead Lake State Park. One narrowly misses the Statue of Liberty and goes on through the north side of Newark International Airport before heading west. The other heads west from Massapequea Preserve, through a high school that has the lowest dropout rate in the country, and is last picked up in Port Elizabeth in Newark Bay.

MASSAPEQUA LEY 1: This east-west ley comes out of the Massapequa Park on Long Island, NY and heads across Parkside Boulevard. If you're looking for a bike workout the park has a fine trail. Across the Boulevard is the Massapequa High School Ames Campus, which claims to have one of the lowest dropout rates in the country. Among its sizable VIP alumni are such folk as actor Alec Baldwin, author Ron Kovic who penned "Born on the Fourth of July," and comedian Jerry Seinfeld.

The school's mission statement includes this great sentence: "We cultivate character by doing what is right even when no one is watching."

Note for Dowsers: Check the area for geospirals. Our rods suggest intense activity.

The ley continues west and passes through the three wings of the Manor Elementary School at Seaford, NY and then makes a track through Hempstead, Jamaica, Brooklyn, crosses Newark Bay to disappear somewhere among the multitudes of shipping containers at the Port Newark-Elizabeth Marine Terminal which in 1985 was the busiest container port in the world. The Terminal is owned by the Port Authority of New York and New Jersey and we found the ley at the McLester and Polaris streets intersection.

MASSAPEQUA LEY 2: This line can be found on the north side of Newark Liberty International Airport on Conrad Road amid United Airlines hangars. The line heads east across Jersey City and touches Liberty Island Sculpture Garden, narrowly missing the Statue of Liberty. The trail is across the Hudson River to the historic Governors Island. If one stands on Division Road intersection facing the main ornate archway leading through Liggett Hall you will be standing on sacred ground where the Native Algonquins talked to their ancestors. They called the place Paggananck meaning Nut Island and it was here they would hunt, fish and what else? — gather nuts, hence the name.

The island is a natural fortress. After the Algonquin departed all who carried guns sought safety lived here: the Dutch, the British, the Colonialists, the US Army and the US Coast Guard. It also served as a prison for Confederate soldiers during the American Civil War.

Strangely, it has an aura of peace that radiates from the ley line and several geospirals that sprinkle various area because the island attracts nearly half a million visitors who come to enjoy its various landscapes and historic buildings and enjoy a variety of uplifting programs each summer season. The current caretakers of the island are the Governors Island Alliance. Visitors can learn more about this historic place at the Alliance's website: Unless you are good at walking on water, you have to take a ferry. The National Parks Service has a page on how to get there. Governors Island links are displayed in the Reference Section.

Meanwhile the ley line sweeps on through Brooklyn and dowsers will find it in The Evergreens Cemetery, which is a beautiful 225 acre area listed on the National Register of Historic Places. It's the last resting place for 73,000 people, 47 of them famous. For instance, the lady who in 1952 wrote the bestseller *Amy Vanderbilt's Complete Book of Etiquette* is buried here. So is Lester "Prez" Young, one of the greatest jazz tenor saxophonists. Back in the days of the big bands he played with Fletcher Henderson, Count Basie and Benny Goodman bands.

Now here's a thing. This ley passes through the chapel at The Evergreens Cemetery. The architect designed the roof with a fully blown four-sided pyramid within the Cosmic Principle and it naturally generates relaxing and healthful energy. What better place to have a pyramid than a cemetery?

The ley continues on along Long Island until it gets to Hempstead Lake, a 67 acre manufactured reservoir created by the Brooklyn Water Supply Company. It is here among the trees on the east side of the water and a few yards north of the Southern State Highway that the two Massapequa leys cross. A marvelous place to simply relax, hang your hat on a branch and stretch out on a blanket and meditate.

The Newark Airport — Liberty Island, Governors Island, Brooklyn ley goes on to a point in the Massapequa Preserve just off Ocean Avenue near the Lake Court intersection and close to the Bethpage Bikeway. Across the park it travels through residential homes before passing through the main body of the Massapequa High School, Main Campus. The ley appears to end a short distance after the school.

FOR DOWSERS : LONG ISLAND LEYS
Coordinates:
Massapequa Ley 1:
Massapequa Park NY.Parkside Blvd. 40°41′08.30″ N 73°27′42.77″ W.
Manor Elementary Sch. Seaford, NY. 40°41′04.39″ N 73°29′07.82″ W
Marine Terminal McLester & Polaris sts. 40°40′03.49″ N 74°09′52.33″ W.

Massapequa Ley 2:
Liberty Airport: Conrad Road. 40°42′22.83″ N 74°10′15.96″ W
Liberty Island Sculpture Gard. 40°41′25.65″ N 74°02′40.66″ W.
Evergreens Cemetery: 40°41′03.76″ N 73°54′01.60″ W.
Massapequa High, Campus 40°40′04.38″ N 73°27′11.40″ W

# PRINCETON: LACED WITH LEYS AND ACADEMICS

rinceton, New Jersey is a community about 50 miles south-west of New York City. It bathes in history, academic accomplishments and is generally a great place to visit, view and photograph. In 2005 Princeton ranked 15th out of a list of 100 towns in the United States in which to "Live and Work" by Money Magazine.

In many ways it reminds one of old England. Perhaps this is because the president of Princeton University in the first part of the 20th Century was one Woodrow Wilson, a radical reformist who possessed strong connections to the United Kingdom and who modeled Princeton on the famous Oxford University. Yes, it is the same Mr. Wilson who went on to be Governor of New Jersey and the 28th President of the United States.

Princeton is also a great place for dowsers to swing a pendulum. The Native Ancestors, the Lenape must have loved the landscape with its abundant meadows and forests, wandering streams and placid lakes because it contains three beautiful and powerful Earth ley lines and an abundance of geospirals. It needs more exploration but it feels close to being a vortex.

This is why visitors who wander along the main Nassau Street are often reluctant to leave. The Earth energies are all powerful and Betty Lou and I discovered them by accident.

We had been invited to see a documentary movie at a leading art gallery in Princeton. "They'll be drinks and eats," said a good friend and that sounded like a cocktail party or a sales mission to which I am both averse. Betty Lou wanted to go and as I did not like the idea of her driving alone on a Saturday night, I reluctantly agreed to go.

But then, something struck me in the shape of a spirit voice: "Princeton: Have you checked for leys, laddie?" Yes, it was Bernard again.

An hour before we left to go, I sat at my laptop and with Google Earth performed a casual scan. Oh, yes! A leyline showed up right on the Nassau Harrison streets intersection — a couple of doors away from the gallery which was our destination. Half an hour later we were on site — and sure enough, the L-rods showed the ley — a strong triple-haired energy.

I had one small glass of wine at the gallery event and next day suffered a hangover. When the research mind cleared, the next few hours on Google Earth showed four leys in Princeton, all with interesting stories. We have named them as the #2 Last Resting Place Ley, the #3 Nassau Street Ley, and #4 the Einstein Ley plus the #1Waldorf Harrison Ley the discovery of which, as I said, came about by sheer accident and led to the finding of the other three. The joy of enquiring dowsing.

# # 1 WALDORF-HARRISON LEY

This ley runs from the teachings of Rudolp Steiner to the creation of color television. It is first picked up some miles north of Princeton in Montgomery County on the Cherry Hill Road. The ley crosses the driveway to the Waldorf School of Princeton. This is one of the international schools whose curriculum is based on the philosophy of noted Austrian philosopher, scientist, educator and esotericist Dr. Rudolph Steiner. In April 1919 while speaking to employees at the Waldorf Astoria factory in war-torn Germany he was asked to establish a school for children of employees.

Dr. Steiner who had just written *The Philosophy of Freedom* agreed but his ideas were radical. He insisted that the complete basic curriculum be made available to all and be independent of political or economic motives to the extent that the law allowed. Also the teachers were to be free to teach according to their best insights into the needs of children and to guide the school in support of its educational goals. In September 1919 the first school opened its doors.

Dr. Steiner stated: "Our highest endeavor must be to develop free human beings who are able of themselves to impart purpose and direction to their lives."

Following Steiner's methology the Princeton School began in 1983 as a playgroup that met in the home of Caroline Phinney and Princeton University professor Bob Phinney. By the following year a full 18-member nursery-kindergarten was established and the school has been built up since then. It now stands on over 20 acres of meadows, woods and a stream. The ley flanks the school on its south-east way to Princeton.

It passes through another place of learning, the Princeton Charter School before heading along Harrison Street's Princeton Shopping Center, then across Nassau Street and on to Lake Carnegie. After crossing the Brunswick Pike otherwise known as US Route 1 it heads into a place that is corporately known as SRI Princeton. In effect it is a place where important technological history was and is still being made.

When David Sarnoff established his research and development center at 201 Washington Road, Princeton just before the attack on Pearl Harbor in 1941, did he have any idea the property was sitting on an ancient ley line and a Native Indian trail? It is not known if Mr. Sarnoff who was the longtime leader of RCA and NBC did in fact choose the property or if the choice was that of a subordinate? Whatever happened, it was a wise decision because the development center created things that changed our world and impacted the lives of most people.

The Princeton site — it is actually located in West Windsor — has scored development credits for such things as the Monochrome-Compatible Electronic Color Television, the first RCA videotape machine, CMOS integrated circuit technology, electron microscopy, the photon-counting photomultiplier, the CCD imager and early optoelectronic components such as lasers and LEDs and in 1968 the invention of the Liquid Crystal Display.

Also in the mid-1950s, while working at the David Sarnoff Research Center, Herbert Kroemer developed key aspects of his theories of hetero-structure physics for which he was a co-recipient of the Nobel Prize in Physics. It has been a power house of invention. We have not had the opportunity of exploring the geospirals abundant in the area.

The ley now heads south-east and crosses another place of learning, the New Horizons Montessori Princeton Junction Campus. This is a method of education that is based on self-directed activity, hands-on learning and collaborative play for younger generations.

The ley's next major crossing point is Success Road at the Colliers Mills Wildlife Management Area (WMA) which covers more than 12,000 acres and is comprised of pitch pine and scrub oak forests, white cedar swamps, fields and lakes and flocks of fascinating birds. The size of the wildlife management area invites exploration and solitude. There are sandy roads and hiking trails awaiting the adventurers. Native Indians used the area for hunting and camping and archaeologists have found flint arrowheads dating back 5,000 years. And if you dowse the ley you will find a great place to sit and meditate in relative silence and perhaps enjoy some lucid dreaming.

We eventually tracked the ley to Maxfield Field, the Lakehurst Naval Air Engineering Station where it disappears.

FOR DOWSERS: Coordinates:
Waldorf School driveway at Princeton NJ 40°24′07.70″ N 74°40′57.87″ W
Nassau and Harrison strs. Intersection 40°21′14.10″ N 74°38′43.45″ W
David Sarnoff SRI Research Unit 40°19′47.15″ N 74°37′38.82″ W
Colliers Mills WMA, Success Rd. 40°04′06.09″ N 74°26′31.55″ W

SPECIAL NOTE FOR NEW LEY HUNTERS: There is an old track energy that could yield some interest for dowsers seeking new leys. It is at Lakehurst Air Station where on May 6th 1937 the German passenger airship LZ 129 Hindenburg caught fire. The zeppelin was to be housed in Hangar #1 which still stands. The ley exists at 40°01′48.12″ N 74°19′01.93″ W a few feet from the main doors before it passes through the building.

# 2 LAST RESTING PLACE LEY:
This Ley starts somewhere north of Princeton and runs south into the urban area passing through the Princeton Regional School District complex, then on to the Princeton Cemetery which is owned by the Nassau Presbyterian Church.

Historians have tagged this last resting place as "The Westminster Abbey of the United States" mainly because of the long list of notables buried here.

If you have seen or heard of the successful Broadway production *Alexander Hamilton*, well, the man who killed him in a duel is buried here. Aaron Burr (1756–1836) was the controversial Revolutionary War hero, politician and third vice president of the United States.

Grover Cleveland (1837–1908) who was the 22nd and 24th president of the United States, along with his wife Frances and their first-born, 13 years old Ruth, the supposed name sake of the Baby Ruth candy bar, are all resting here side by side. The afternoon we visited the cemetery we found a fresh large wreath had been placed on the Cleveland gravestone along with a United States flag and some white necklaces. Tim, the cemetery director told us that every March 18th in the morning a military and civilian memorial service is held at the grave side and a new wreath is placed.

Close by we discovered the grave markers of John and Katherine O'Hara. John wrote such best sellers as *Appointment in Samarra, Ten North Frederick* and *Pal Joey*. Across the way is the last resting place of Helen Dukas who was Albert Einstein's personal secretary for 28 years.

You may have heard of the Gallup Polls. George Gallup, statistician and journalist and pioneer in public opinion and market research is buried here in Princeton.

Some folks would have thought that Paul Robeson who was born in Princeton would have been buried here. Athlete, actor, singer, Civil Rights activist, he died in Philadelphia and was buried in Westchester County, NY. Still, his parents William and Maria Robeson who called Princeton home are buried in the Cemetery. When the great man died in 1976 the citizens of the Princeton named a street after him. Paul Robeson Place.

There are many stories one could tell of great people buried in Princeton.

Among the distinguished academics there are also generals, composers, philosophers, financiers, murder victims, mathematicians, engineers, inventors, war heroes and signers of the Declaration of Independence such as John Witherspoon (1723–1794).

The Ley can be found coming southbound out of the cemetery on Higgins-North Tulane intersection. After following South Tulane St. the Ley crosses Nassau St. and enters Princeton University. Paralleling Chancellor Way, it first passes through the University's Firestone Library, flanks the west end of the Chapel, touches the Department of English, then passes through the gardens of the School of Architecture, then travels between Prospect House and the Department of Music before heading straight through the Department of East Asian Studies.

It is next found on the playing field at Roberts Stadium before passing through the south-west end of the University Boathouse, home to Princeton Rowing Teams, on the human-made Lake Carnegie, a gift of Andrew Carnegie. The ley crosses Brunswick Pike / US Route 1 at the railway overpass and indeed the ley and the rails are together until both reach the Princeton Junction/Amtrak mainline railway station.

FOR DOWSERS:
Pr.Cemetery / Higgins St: 40°21′09.04″ N 74°39′33.81″ W.
Nassau S. Tulane intersect: 40°21′00.31″ N 74°39′28.43″ W
Princeton Boathouse: 40°20′21.07″ N 74°39′02.82″ W
US Route 1 at Rail Overpass: 40°19′45.01″ N 74°38′22.91″ W
Amtrak / Princeton Junction: 40°18′59.08″ N 74°37′23.70″ W

#3 NASSAU STREET LEY
From The Jewish Center to Global Education
This leyline is on an east-west course and is picked up in the grounds of The Jewish Center of Princeton on the south side parking area and generally runs parallel to Nassau Street but in an ever decreasing closeness. It crosses Harrison and by the time it reaches Washington St. it is starting to cross Nassau. Carry a pendulum and you will find it on the island sidewalk at the entrance to Palmer Square.

The ley moves on to the Princeton Battle Monument which reminds the visitor of that day January 3, 1777 when the peaceful winter fields and woods near Princeton — now Battlefield Park — were transformed into what historians say was the fiercest and bloodiest fight of its size during the American Revolution.

During this critical battle, American troops under General George Washington surprised and defeated a force of British Regulars. It came at the end of ten crucial days which saw the celebrated Christmas night crossing of the Delaware River and two battles in Trenton. The Battle of Princeton gave Washington his first victory against the British Regulars. At one time the battle moved over a mile away to the College of New Jersey which is now Princeton University.

From the Battle Monument the ley swings through Morven, once the official residence of the governor of New Jersey. It is now known officially as Morven Museum & Garden, a historic 18th-century house at 55 Stockton Street in Princeton.

The Nassau Street Ley next appears at a fascinating and unique complex at 660 Rosedale Road. Located in a distinctive saucer-shaped meadow the Educational Testing Service (ETS), was founded in 1947 and is the world's largest private nonprofit educational testing and assessment organization. In total, ETS annually administers 20 million exams in the U.S. and in 180 other countries. In actuality they operate in Lawrence Township, but run with a Princeton address. You may like the line on their website: "At ETS, we recruit people who love learning and teaching and strive to maintain the highest standards in the field of education."

The Nassau Street Ley can be found running across the driveway into the Lord Hall building then through the Chauncey Conference Center. It continues on across New Jersey towards Hopewell which we have not tracked at this time.

FOR DOWSERS: The coordinates of this ley are:
The Jewish Center on Nassau St: 40°21′18.54″ N 74°38′25.40″ W
Nassau St/Palmer Square: 40°20′58.28″ N 74°39′51.44″ W
Educational Testing Service: 40°20′39.55″ N 74°42′46.13″ W

#4 THE EINSTEIN LEY
If a dowser had been visiting south-west Princeton in the 1940s and early 1950s, before urbanization had spread into the suburbs, he or she would likely have seen an elderly man with a mop of graying hair, attired in a heavy woolen overcoat walking to work. Historians say he sometimes got lost, but mostly he made tracks to his office tucked away in a stately

looking Edwardian building made even more majestic because it has an elegant tower reaching for the sky.

The man's name was Albert Einstein and the building, Fuld Hall was and is home to some of the most powerful forward thinkers in the world. In fact this has been the case since the Institute for Advanced Studies was created in 1930 by American educator Abraham Flexner, together with philanthropists Louis Bamberger and Caroline Bamberger Fuld.

In those early days the boffins had temporary offices in Princeton University's Fine Hall with the mathematics people until Fuld Hall was completed in the meadows adjoining Battlefield Park. Flexner brought together some of the greatest minds in history to collaborate on intellectual discovery and research in Princeton.

Distinguished scientists and scholars such as logician and philosopher Kurt Gödel; J. Robert Oppenheimer of the Manhattan Project; iconologist Erwin Panofsky; archaeologist and first woman member of the Institute Hetty Goldman; archaeologist in ancient Greco Studies Homer A. Thompson; mathematician and specialist in Quantum Mechanics John von Neumann; diplomat, political scientist and historian George Kennan; mathematician, theoretical physicist and philosopher Hermann Weyl; and anthropologist known for Interpretation of Cultures Clifford Geertz.

Albert Einstein joined the Institute as a professor of theoretical physics in 1933 and made the town his academic home for over 20 years. It was here he worked on nagging questions remaining from his Special Theory (1905) and General Theory of Relativity(1915). Questions concerned his thinking about light, gravity and acceleration and the opening of an entirely new field in Physics. This had happened earlier in 1919 when a British astronomer actually proved a critical element in the theory which made the German-born scientist an immediate celebrity.

Einstein and wife Elsa fled Germany in 1933 as Nazism reared its ugly head and settled in Princeton. In 1935 they moved into the newly built home at 112 Mercer Street where he lived until he died on April 18th 1955.

One wonders if all the many times he walked the half a mile to his office at the Institute did he ever think or feel that the building was situated on a special energy, a triple-haired ley with an abundance of leys surrounding the place? As we have seen many times leys and their often accompanying geospirals inspire creative thought, good working and studying environments, healthy living and positive motivation.

Perhaps, Dr. Einstein's consciousness was on a different vibration, who knows? It would be interesting to know with all the acreage then available why Abraham Flexner and his companions selected to build the Institute for Advanced Studies on a vibrant triple-haired ley.

Did Abraham Flexner stand in that Princeton meadow almost 90 years ago and simply say: "Intuitively I feel this is the site for our Institute. It feels right." Or did he find a dowser among his associates and friends who demonstrated that this was indeed the right place.

It was another age when dowsing or "witching" as the religionists termed it, was still very much hidden on Main Street, America, so we might safely conclude Abraham Flexner intuited the point of location. Indeed, it was the right decision.

The energy track of the Einstein Ley is first found at Littlebrook School in north-east Princeton and it starts on a south-west route. It actually crosses all three other Princeton leys and in doing so crosses through the Harrison Street Park, Powers Field at Princeton University Stadium that replaced the old Palmer Stadium, then through the Department of Physics and onto the Springdale Golf Course originally the Princeton Golf Club which dates back to the 1890s and was formed by alumni, faculty and undergraduates. The name was changed in 1922.

The ley moves onto Einstein Drive where at #1 is the Institute for Advance Studies. It passes across the front of the building then continues south-west across the Princeton Battlefield Park, along the Princeton Pike which was originally a Lenape trail. It then goes on to another place of advanced learning, the Chapin Private School close to where the Pike crosses Province Line Road.

The Einstein Ley is a line that reflects education from almost beginning to end. The lesson here is: If you want to build a place for innovative thinkers and action, find a ley line amid a collection of geospirals. Princeton Ley is a fine example.

FOR DOWSERS
Einstein Ley coordinates:
Littlebrook School: 40°21′49.39" N 74°38′17.91" W
Harrison Park: 40°21′11.40" N 74°38′41.69" W
Princeton U. Stadium: 40°20′46.06" N 74°39′00.87" W
Ins for Advanced Studies: 40°19′55.22" N 74°40′04.99" W
Chapin School: 40°18′35.99" N 74°41′37.48" W
PRINCETON NJ NOTES

NOTE ONE: Cuyler Hall on Elm Drive in Princeton contains 50 rooms on four floors for students and the forecourt presents an opportunity to test the Cosmic Principle at work. The pathways form a complete square with center paths forming a diagonal cross. An irresistible attraction. Holding a pendulum loosely at my side I walked along a path and as I reached the cross the pendulum started swinging vigorously — counter clockwise. The pendulum refused a clockwise spin. An excellent Cosmic Principle! What a delight. If you are a student or a visitor, stop on the forecourt and enjoy the relaxing aura. It is beautiful. If you have a pendulum try it out on the cross.

NOTE TWO: Opportunity for work on another ley. Three miles south-east of Princeton there is evidence of ley activity at Grovers Mill Pond and the adjoining Van Nest Park on the Cranbury Road. According to Orson Welles this was the landing place for the Martians in his 1937 radio drama "The War of the Worlds" which triggered widespread concern and occasional panic. In the park there is a monument commemorating the actor-producer-writer and the landing. Incidentally the park is a great place to relax mainly because of the ley but also the many geospirals. For ley seekers the coordinates are: 40°18′46.81" N 74°36′16.95".

# THE WILD BIRD OASIS LEY

When cosmic energy manipulators on the Other Side get together to make something known it is truly amazing how they accomplish this without a dowser feeling he or she is being manipulated. How we found this next ley is "auto-dowsing" when unbeknown to a person's conscious mind, the higher consciousness decides to dowse on its own.

In late February 2016 while researching this book, I conducted a metaphysical development class at our home base in Pemberton. A lady named Doris told me of a shop in Medford Lakes, New Jersey that deals in birdseed but also has crystals, pendulums and some pyramids.

Pyramids? The word caught my attention. Next morning Betty Lou and I found ourselves outside a store with a huge sign: "A Wild Bird Oasis: A Place for Wild Birds and Nature Lovers."

Over the years I have developed a mild suspicion about New Age stores and although this one did not specifically look like it, I still did not feel totally interested. Pyramids in a bird seed shop? But Betty Lou loves birds, so in we went and found enough bird seed to keep a flock fed for a hundred years. I searched for a Himalayan salt pyramid mentioned by Doris but they were sold. Still they had some fascinating bird houses with pyramid tops — and yes, Betty Lou's pendulum spun counter-clockwise as usual.

A healthy looking and picturesque creek runs behind the store and owners Hank and Linda Wright have birdhouses outside a window and high over the water where Red Cardinals, Blue Jays and other birds came visiting and feeding.

Among various ceramic pots, bird signs, bird pictures, and fascinating bits and pieces we found some crystals. Betty Lou wanted an amethyst so I suggested she use her pendulum to select the right one. This she did and then started talking with Linda the owner.

"Please hold my pendulum," she called out.

Taking it, I stood patiently nearby arms at my side with one of my hands casually holding the pendulum's chain. It was then I noticed an unusual quiet. My hand was not moving but the pendulum was indeed swinging. Amazed, I stared but did nothing but let it swing. It went round faster and faster. Then I realized it was exactly the same sort of swing that happens when I stand on a ley line.

"Betty Lou," I said trying to stay casual. "Guess what? There's a leyline passing through this shop."

Immediately the two came over and Betty Lou started explaining about earth energies and ley lines to Linda. My L-rods were in the car outside and I fetched them. They showed a ley crossing the store.

Linda listened then asked various questions and I told her about geospirals and their relaxing and healing energies. "Let's see if there is one here," I said putting one rod into the search mode.

It swung round to face the large window at the front of the store. I walked towards the window and within six inches of the glass the rod swung into reverse. "You also have a geospiral in the shop," I said. "Do people come in to browse and stay? Like they just want to hang out?"

"Oh, yes," replied Linda with a puzzled smile. "They do it quite often."

We showed her where to place a chair on the ley which was also well within the geospiral's Area of Influence. "If you ever need a shot of rejuvenating energy to calm your mind, perhaps heal some aches or tiredness, just sit in this chair for 20 minutes and you'll feel the difference."

Outside Betty Lou and I sat in the car. "That whole thing was weird. From the moment Doris told me about this place, I simply had to come. Now I know why. The Cosmic Forces want us to know about this ley."

We are calling this the Wild Birds Oasis Ley because that is where we found it. The ley line stretches almost east-west and vice versa across New Jersey. From Medford Lakes east the line goes to Tabernacle Township where it passes directly through the very active Seneca High School which has 1,229 students with 113 full time teachers. According to a US News report students have an incredible 98% proficiency in language.

The ley continues across the state and heads through a flotilla of big and small boats at Forked River before heading out into the Atlantic.

Meanwhile, heading west from Medford Lakes the line runs through the Arrowhead Tennis Club and passes through a number of communities including Bellmawr, the Eagle Point oil refinery at Westville, a community called National Park and another called Thoroughfare. We pause here because the ley serves an intriguing place originally known as Sanitarium Playground but now Soupy Island.

Every year during the summer children from all walks of life are invited to Soupy Island to get some free family fun and a free meal of soup, crackers and milk. Here is a true vintage playground with lots of swings, covered picnic tables, swimming pools including a childrens' wading pool, a fully sized 19th century carousel with magnificent horses and a fabulous covered slide built in 1907.

The Wild Bird Oasis Ley passes right by the slide and even when the place is deserted like in the winter months, if you are quiet you can still hear the sounds of children laughing in fact lots of laughing.

And if you notice tinges of sadness that is because Soupy Island originated in times of frantic hope and heavy sadness. A time when the kid you made friends with last year no longer comes to play.

As we saw with The Saranac Ley, tuberculosis or "consumption" was rampant in the middle to later years of the 19th century. No one possessed a cure but doctors advised the afflicted to get out of the cities and seek fresh air. That was the goal of The Sanitarium Association created in 1877 by amusement park owner, John F. Smith to help suffering children. The project was promptly joined by Philadelphia and Camden philanthropists and volunteers including many doctors. Originally on an island they were forced to move when the Delaware River was widened and the island wiped out. Smith chose the present location at Red Bank, a piece of wooded land with a beach front on the Delaware.

Did Mr. Smith or any of the doctors and volunteers know that they could not have selected a better place? It provided not only fresh air and the close proximity of the tides bringing invigorating sea energy, it was on two ley lines, the Wild Bird Oasis Ley and the William Penn Ley that comes from Philadelphia and a variety of geospirals.

It's little wonder that when children and adults come to Soupy Island today, there is a feeling of wanting to stay. It's the extensive aura of Yin energy — healing and relaxing.

When Sanitariums started closing in the 1960s the directors on Soupy Island decided to continue with their loving service to children: a bowl of soup, snacks, milk, and crackers This tradition still continues today in the original soup kitchen.

Sure there is a mixture of energies at Soupy Island. You can feel and sometimes hear them. Nature intended the place for healing, love and comfort.

When Betty Lou and I visited the place on a chilly winter's afternoon, she told me: "I don't like the place. I feel as if I had to get away from the sadness." When we arrived home and brought up the story of the Sanitarium Playground she said: "We're going to go back. I want to go back there." That's the power of all the different energies there.

As we were leaving the playground, a voice whispered in my ear: "Robert, we were here too. It was always a special place for our people too."

"Who are you?"

"The Lenape Nation."

# FORT MIFFLIN – GHOSTS OF THE PAST

The Wild Birds Oasis Ley leaves Soupy island and crosses the Delaware River into Pennsylvania.

Every day thousands of people pass over an ancient fortification known as Fort Mifflin and unless you know it exists are never conscious of the fact. Aircraft from all over the States and the Earth skim over the battlements at 300 feet as they prepare to land at Philadelphia International Airport.

Ancient? Fort Mifflin is the only military base in use that is older than the nation itself. In 1962, the federal government deeded Fort Mifflin to the City of Philadelphia. However part of Fort Mifflin remains an active base for the United States Army Corp of Engineers which makes it the oldest active military base in the United States and the only base in use that pre-dates the Declaration of Independence.

It is also on the western leg of the Wild Bird Oasis Ley which adds to the Fort's great attraction for school students, tourists, ghost hunters and their kin.

The Fort's historical legacy goes deeper and its origins seem to be buried in history. The site commands an excellent view of the Delaware River and it is highly likely our Native Ancestors were not only aware but used it as well.

Fort Mifflin, originally called Fort Island Battery and known later as Mud Island Fort, was commissioned in 1771 and sits on Mud Island on the Delaware River near Philadelphia International Airport.

In the fall of 1777 General Washington's Army was aiming for Valley Forge, Pennsylvania where they would spend the winter. The British forces were sandwiched between as they occupied Philadelphia. On the Delaware River 400 American troops stationed at Fort Mifflin effectively blocked the waterway and frustrated British naval attempts to re-supply beleaguered forces in the city. Spasmodic fighting continued for six weeks.

At daybreak on November 10, 1777, the British fleet launched a naval attack. Cannon fire rained down on Fort Mifflin in what became known as the largest bombardment of the Revolutionary War. Some historians say during one hour over 1,000 cannon balls landed on the Fort. That's a blast every 3.6 seconds. The battle lasted five days in atrociously stormy weather and high tides. Finally, the American soldiers, their ammunition and food supplies depleted, slipped through the night to safety across the Delaware while a 40-man contingent burned and razed the old Fort.

The valiant efforts of the American soldiers at Fort Mifflin held the British Navy at bay in order to give Washington and his troops time to arrive safely at Valley Forge where they shaped a strong and efficient army. They crossed the Delaware at Trenton on Christmas Day.

During that winter, Washington commissioned a French-born architect, serving as an officer with the engineers at Valley Forge, to design a new Fort Mifflin. The Frenchman's name was Pierre L'Enfant and his plans, based on European styles — mostly French and Venetian — can be seen today in real life. The plans were actually implemented at Mifflin by another Frenchman artillerist who served in the American Army, Louis de Tousard. He authored two very influential books: one that became the blueprint for West Point and the other an artillery officers' manual that became standard in the young US Army.

But it is Pierre L'Enfant who sparks our dowser's attention for what will become obvious. After the Revolutionary War was over, L'enfant started an architectural practice in New York City but George Washington called again. This time it was for L'Enfant to convert the Old City Hall in New York to Federal Hall to serve the new U.S. Congress. Then the President called again. "We need an architectural plan for a new city." That city became Washington DC.

# PIERRE L'ENFANT — A MAN WHO KNEW THE ENERGY

Pierre — he really called himself Peter — perhaps because he was a Catholic, perhaps because he wanted to seem American, perhaps he did not like a French first name. Qui sait? Who knows ?

One warm day in March with the New Jersey skies a clear sunny blue Betty Lou and I ventured out to historic Fort Mifflin, a site hidden away close to the landing strip at Philadelphia airport. The Fort's mitigating factor is that the building overlooks the wide expanse of the Delaware River and one can easily imagine an historic battle taking place here. It almost resembles a movie set — dramatic! Several 18th century cannon and a stumpy but ornate mortar greet those who venture within its battlements.

Our first hint of something peculiar occurred when a thin, bespectacled man carrying a metal box and wearing a tight headset emerged from a darkened tunnel that echoed and felt damp.

"Paranormal," he whispered. "Ghost hunting," he added as if he had to apologize. Before we could ask if he had caught anything, he slid silently away into the darkness.

We wandered through the old brick buildings, a mess hall, sleeping quarters for 400 men. To be honest we could not imagine so many soldiers in such cramped places. Perhaps two centuries ago they were all small in stature. The commandant's house is still there and one can easily imagine him coming out to inspect the troops lined up outside.

Our mission was two-fold. One to take photographs and two, check the ley line that runs through the west end of Fort Mifflin. As one climbs the steps to the top of the great walls the layout is impressive. The battlements are so designed that if ever there might be an attempt by infantry to scale the bastions there would be no cover and all invaders could be shot down quite easily. The bastions were built in arrowhead formations and defense forces manning the positions possessed excellent views of adjoining walls and any invaders approaching.

Fort Mifflin reminded me of similar bastions built by the Venetians at Nicosia and Famagsta on the Mediterranean island of Cyprus early in the 16th century. Both failed after prolonged sieges by the Ottoman Turks, but not because of the bastion design but lack of food and water.

As I stood on the bastion with the ley under my feet, my thoughts seemed to bother a spirit that sounded close by.

"No! No! No!"

The voice was squeaky and dramatic and a far cry from the cultured and modulated Oxford tone used by Bernard. "Who's this?"

"Mon Dieu! The design is mine. It is a modication of the plans laid out by the master architect Leonardo da Vinci. The Venetians had nothing to do with it. Rein! You understand?"

"You made your point, sir," I said, then holding my camera as if to take a photo, I remarked: "I'm standing on a ley line, you know that don't you?"

"Line? Oh, oui! La ligne ley!" exclaimed the voice rising an octave with undisguised happiness. "La ligne ley! You know?"

"Yes, I have walked many ligne leys," I said. "I find them with the L-rods."

"Your friend, Thomas Passey, he was un chercheur de ligne like you."

Tom was the dowsing master from my days in British Columbia. Since working on this book I have felt him around particularly when on field trips and when writing difficult descriptions, the words simply come to mind as if my brain is speared by an arrow.

"Monsieur Tom says for me to tell you — Hurry up! Stop wasting time on research."

Shaking my head I said: "Peter...is that your name?" It was a guess.

"Simply ask the question that is on your mind."

It was blunt. "When and where did you become un chercheur de ligne — a ley line hunter? A dowser?"

"A l'académie de Paris," he said. "When I studied architecture and art - there was a student there whose father practiced radiesthésie. You understand ? That is a healing modalité using le pendule — you know? The pendulum?"

Betty Lou approached. "Who are you talking to?"

"A fellow named Peter. "Sounds like Pierre l'Enfant who designed these battlements."

Peter ignored the interruption. His conscious was still back to his youth in Paris. "The father would occasionally take us out into the forests for — hunting, that is water and many things. He would search for coal, relics from antiquity. The father used small branches from trees and also the pendulum," he said, then lowering his tone he added: "Father warned us not to disclose this to anybody," he said with a shrug, "because we could be executed, burned, placed in prison for practicing la magie — the magic."

"Witchcraft," I said. "This was before the Revolution?"

"Bien sûr! Of course! But we all knew it was coming so that's when I came to America."

The energy was floating in front of me and it seemed to get bigger and more intense. "La ville de Washington! You know there is une grande ligne ley?"

I nodded.

A torrent of words smashed through the ether, a mix of two languages, English and French, trying to explain how he and George Washington created the layout for what would be the federal capitol of America. One had the impression that l'Enfant's major stumbling block was the lingering English traditional small thinking still dominant in America and the fact the government was not only reluctant to pay his bills and salary but failed him miserably.

Peter kept talking about his vision for the "grande promenade publique " which translated meant the National Mall where everyone, aristocrat and worker alike walked shoulder to shoulder in total equality.

"You know there is a triple-haired ley line existing along the middle of the National Mall?"

"Oh oui, bien sûr! " he exclaimed, then blurted out in great excitement, "That is why the Mall is there. The energie is bon — good, eh?" For a few moments he laughed. "When all is quiet there, I take my friends for walks along the promenade. No one sees us, except perhaps the children. Les enfants — they see us but their parents inform them they are liars."

His laughter seemed to echo across the battlements as he faded. I have often wondered what would happen if all the spirits who wander around the National Mall suddenly appeared to all and sundry. That would tickle Monsieur Peter l'Enfant for sure.

As Betty Lou and I started to leave Fort Mifflin the ghost hunter reappeared from a dark tunnel. "Did you find anything?" I enquired.

The man shook his head. "Not today."

"Try the west battlements. Spirits like the sun and fresh air up there," I said.

Then as we drove home, I said: "We must take a look at Washington, DC."

FOR DOWSERS:
The Wild Bird Oasis Ley. Coordinates:
Forked River NJ: E. Lacey & Davenport 39°49'49.74" N 74°11'05.91" W
Seneca High, Tabernacle NJ 39°51'28.49" N 74°43'05.54" W
The Wild Bird Oasis, Medford Lakes NJ 39°51'55.71" N 74°48'27.00" W
Soupy Island, West Deptford NJ 39°52'32.41" N 75°10'39.58" W
Historic Fort Mifflin, PA. 39°52'34.38" N 75°12'47.50" W
Phil. Air. Term B/Depart. Rd: 39°52'35.41" N 75°14'36.52" W

Note: There is evidence of a second ley line at Philadelphia Airport's Terminal F also on the Departures Road.

# DOWSING THE NATIONAL MALL LEY

Washington is an amazing city. Pick up a city map or browse over to Google Earth and bring up Washington, DC. The design of the grid system has brought compliments and praise from various parts of the world. John W. Reps is Professor Emeritus Department of City and Regional Planning, Cornell University at Ithaca, NY.

In his book *The Making of Urban America: A History of City Planning in the United States,* he writes: *"Certainly in its magnitude, its clever fitting of a generally symmetrical design to irregular topography and its generous provision for a variety of open spaces, the plan for Washington must stand as one of the great city planning efforts of all time."*

The next time you get a chance to spend a day in Washington DC take your dowsing instruments and head for the Washington Monument. It looks like an Egyptian obelisk but it is not. It is a "Made in the USA" needle. It does however perform two impressive functions.

It conforms and functions to the Cosmic Principle and it stands on a powerful ley line that runs through the US Capitol building, the seat of Government and then cuts a line along the middle of the National Mall.

A dowser can have tremendous and gratifying experiences exploring or even taking some kids or open-minded adults along and showing them the power centers that grace the United States national scene.

First the obelisk. Its proper name is the Washington Monument, an obelisk built to commemorate George Washington, once commander-in-chief of the Continental Army and the first American president. This obelisk is made of marble, granite and bluestone gneiss a foliated metamorphic rock.

It stands 555 feet and as such is the tallest obelisk in the world.

Building the Monument was no easy and short-lived task. Construction began in 1848 and was halted in 1854 for three years due to a lack of funds mainly from a struggle for control over the Washington National Monument Society and the intervention of the American Civil War.

The stone structure was completed in 1884, but internal ironwork, the knoll, and other finishing touches were not completed until 1888. An eagle-eyed observer may notice differences in the color of marble stone, the result of different sources at different times.

Designed by architect Robert Mills, the original monument had four sides but a flat top — depriving it of its true pyramidal status and power. Eventually Mills changed it to a pointed marble pyramidion in 1884. The cornerstone was laid on July 4, 1848; the first stone at the 152-foot level was laid August 7, 1880, the capstone was set on December 6, 1884, and the completed monument was dedicated on February 21, 1885. As pilgrims following the Cosmic Principle know, it is the capstone that gives the pyramid and obelisk its cosmic power.

Officially opened on October 9, 1888 it became the world's tallest structure, a title previously held by the Cologne Cathedral. The monument held this designation until 1889, when the Eiffel Tower was completed in Paris, France.

The monument was damaged during the 2011 Virginia earthquake and Hurricane Irene in the same year and remained closed to the public for over two and a half years for repairs. The National Park Service and the Trust for the National Mall reopened the Washington Monument to visitors in May 2014.

Its Area of Influence can be felt and dowsed at Constitution Avenue on the north side and Independence Avenue on the south side which means the park is a great place to relax, let go of stress and feel the healing benefits of the Cosmos.

As they say in the commercials: But wait, there's more. A triple-haired ley line breaks right through the Washington Monument. Here is its route.

On a close to east-west axis, the ley comes in through the Robert F. Kennedy Stadium, along East Capitol Street NE and Lincoln Park, sweeps through the United States Capitol building and the Ulysses S. Grant Memorial. It heads east in this order, the Capitol Reflecting Pool, the National Mall, Washington Monument, the World War II Memorial and and the Lincoln Memorial. Continuing East it crosses the Potomac River to the northern part of the Arlington National Cemtery.

There's more. Two single haired leys one on a north-west to south-east course crosses the Senate in the Capitol Building, the other on a north-south course crosses both chambers, the US Senate and the US House of Representatives including the Capitol Dome in between.

In addition there are several blind springs giving off at least 17 geo-spirals making the Capitol Building area a great place for attracting men and women with various creative and organizational talents and skills. It is also a region, a vortex that encourages and manifests healing, wellbeing and a state of higher consciousness.

Great stuff, Pierre! Une magnifique ligne!

Before we leave. Mention was made of the ley running through Arlington National Cemetery and thereby hangs a story.

Peter L'Enfant, born in Paris, France, August 2nd 1754 was a lively Leo, a visionary genius at planning, died in poverty on June 14th, 1825. Buried on the Digges Farm, also known as Green Hill, Prince Georges County, Maryland. Historians say he left behind three watches, three compasses, some books, some maps, and surveying instruments, whose total value was about forty-five dollars.

Almost a hundred years were to pass before people in high places realized one of the Nation's great architects was buried in an obscure farm in Maryland. On April 19, 1909, the adjutant general of the War Department ordered the disinterment. L'Enfant's remains were placed in a metal-lined casket, draped with the American flag and moved to Mount Olivet Cemetery, Washington D.C. On April 28, 1909 a military escort conveyed the remains to the U.S. Capitol Building where they lay in state for three hours. They were then taken by military escort to Arlington National Cemetery. There, in front of the Mansion, they were reinterred at a special site. A special act of Congress directed the erection of a monument at the grave.

On the afternoon of May 22, 1911, the monument marking the grave of Pierre Charles L'Enfant was dedicated. The service took place on the portico of the Arlington House, where chairs had been arranged to make a miniature open-air theater. The monument was draped with the American flag. It was so arranged that all those attending the dedication saw the memorial monument and the great city he designed stretched out in all its glory aided by a triple-haired ley and an abundance of geospirals.

His spirit must have danced ecstatically on top of the monument because all he sought was recognition in lieu of cash, even if it took 85 years or so. But those who saw him would not tell. It was not the done thing.

"La ville de Washington! You know there is une grande ligne ley?"

FOR DOWSERS: The National Mall Ley
Robert F. Kennedy Stadium: 38°53′24.95″ N 76°58′18.82″ W
Fountain, US Capitol Building: 38°53′23.38″ N 77°00′36.65″ W
The Washington Monument: 38°53′23.10″ N 77°02′07.91″ W
US Marine Corps Mem. Park: 38°53′19.83″ N 77°04′09.91″ W

Note 1: Look for an additional ley crossing the US Marine Corps Park from south-west to north-east and passing through the Iwo Jima Memorial at 38°53′25.50″ N 77°04′10.97″ W

Note 2: Pierre L'Enfant Memorial, at Arlington National Cemetery. 38°52′51.92″ N 77°04′20.16″ W

# THE WILLIAM PENN LEY

Philadelphia, Pennsylvania is a mere 100 miles from New York City and 130 miles from Washington, D.C., and a whole lot of Philadelphians like to think they are in the center if not the middle of everything. The City of Brotherly Love has a lot to show off the top: Independence Hall where the Consititution was signed, that historic symbol of freedom the Liberty Bell and the Philadelphia Museum of Art and its famous 72 steps featured in the movie "Rocky." Did someone say 72 steps? That reduces to nine again. The museum has no leys but it does bathe in a whole nest of geospirals gushing Yin energy,

Philadelphia contains two impressive leys that form a complete cross, straight enough for some to cry "A Christian city!" One triple-haired ley runs 13 miles down an entire street. Countless thousands of people cross over it every day, and a whole lot of people rely on its relaxing, uplifting energy for business, studies and recuperation. The other ley even contains a large pyramid fitting the Cosmic Principle. Both leys are accompanied by numerous educational, artistic, spiritual, relaxing and health related activies.

The two leys cross each other at City Hall which was the plan and the dream of William Penn. It is difficult to say that this esteemed Quaker, this great entrepeneur from England had no idea of what he was doing when he created the essence, the basic plan of Philadephia. Of course he knew. The city could not have been built around a better more dynamic Cosmic energy force.

An observer standing on either North or South Broad Street looking towards the city center will spot a large building appearing to block the way. That for the uninitiated is Philadelphia's City Hall. It is the largest such building in the United States with almost 700 rooms towering, it seems, to the sky with a human figure standing precariously on top.

This is William Penn. Various people have expressed desires over the years to kidnap it or buy it to put in their backyard but it is no mere statue. It stands 37 feet tall, made of bronze and weighs 27 tons. It is said to be the tallest statue standing on the top of any building in the world. Yes, Mr. Penn looks down from a tower some 500 feet up.

The ley runs along the sidewalk on the west side of North Broad and the center and east side if you are on South Broad Street.

Before we get involved in the ley and its impact on the community let us tune in with some history.

The son of an admiral, William Penn was born in London, England in October 1644 and grew up to be a real estate entrepreneur, philosopher, an active Quaker and a vociferous high spirited agitator for religious freedom. This was the era of Puritans, Oliver Cromwell and the sobering beheading of a British monarch, King Charles the First.

In 1681, Charles II of England granted William Penn a charter for what would become the Pennsylvania colony. Although awarded by royal charter Penn purchased the land from the Lenapes to stay on good terms with the Native Americans in the hope of ensuring peace for his colony. Penn named the growing community Philadelphia, which is Greek for brotherly love stemming from philos meaning "friendship" and adelphos meaning "brother." As a Quaker, Penn had experienced severe religious persecution in England, an outfalling of the Protestant versus Catholic wars that gripped western Europe and the Isles. Penn wanted his colony to be a place where anyone could worship freely, be more spiritual, an attitude that also appealed to Native Indians.

Penn hoped the new community would serve more like an English town with a rural countryside and its proximity to the Delaware River provided an opportunity to serve as a port and place for government.

History says that Penn laid out Philadelphia streets and roads on a grid plan to keep houses and businesses spread far apart, with areas for gardens and orchards. It was a grid based on natural Earth energy. Both Quakers and Masons were well aware of divining, another name for dowsing, but practiced the art covertly because of witch trials that were rampant in some of the new colonies, notably Connecticut — 1647 to 1697.

So Philadelphia has a long 13 mile arterial street that manifests positive Earth energies from a triple-haired ley. This phenomenon is flanked by spring-based geospirals which collectively add to the power. Remember, each ley comes with a lateral and vertical Area of Influence. Broad Street is a powerhouse of Earth energy. A master stroke of planning.

But was it by accident? Was it by coincidence? Or did the original father, or his cohorts, know and planned the route because of the Earth and its beneficial energies?.

Today, North Broad Street is dotted with churches, spiritual healing centers, tabernacles, synagogues and temples. For instance the beautiful statuesque Masonic Temple is at 1 North Broad St, a stone throw from City Hall. Masons never do anything accidentally.

Starting in 1925 the tall white building at 400 North Broad was once home to the great Philadelphia Inquirer newspaper and some oustanding awarding-winning journalists. In fact during the 1970s and '80s under the leadership of Gene Roberts it reaped 17 Pulitzer Prizes. Investgative jouralists Donald L Bartlett and James B. Steele won Pulitizers and various other awards while at the Inquirer before moving on to Time Magazine.

The building was sold in 2011 and the newspaper moved out of the Broad Street energy zone. In 2015 the purchaser Bart Blatstein said he would attempt to turn the edifice into a 125 room boutique hotel.

The Pennsylvania Academy of the Fine Arts is a museum and art school founded in 1805. It is the first and oldest art museum and art school in the United States. You will find it among the Earth energies of North Broad.

From West Oxford Avenue intersection for at least three city blocks on both sides of the street the sightseeing dowser will witness tall, hefty buildings, doctors, nurses, lab technicians, students, milling around the sidewalks, mini-parks and alcoves. This is the hallowed ground of a university hospital. Once upon a time it was not like this at all.

Russell Herman Conwell (1843 –1925) started life as a soldier in the Civil War with the Union Army. With the "Mountain Boys" of Masschusetts he became known as a hero, never leaving any soldier behind. Later he became an American Baptist minister, orator, philan-thropist, lawyer and writer, in fact he wrote a life-changing classic which is still in the bookstores (and Amazon) today. It is frequently quoted in national self-improvement workshops and lectures. The title? *Acres of Diamonds.*

Reverend Conwell possessed a goal, an ambition to see a college and throughout the 1880s in Philadelphia he started teaching his writings, first to a couple of students, then six, then as word travelled the classes prompted the need for an established school.

On January 18, 1892 a three-story house at 3403 North Broad was purchased and re-named Samaritan Hospital. Dr. Conwell was appointed president of the 20-bed hospital, which came with a mission: to provide free care for those unable to afford payment, regardless of race, nation-ality or creed.

Today, that house only exists in photos and memories. In its place is Temple University with its big T logo that stands out on a set of buildings along North Broad. The university has 37,000 students, 31,000 full time and offers an incredible array of subjects.

The actual site where the three-story house number 3403 North Broad actually stood 124 years ago, has given way to a nine story building that takes up much of the block. Now the address is 3401 North Broad, Temple University Hospital. But this is only a part.

Across the street is another nine story building, strangely designed with no windows. It is truly weird, until someone points out it is Temple's Medical Research Building. Further along the street is Lewis Katz School of Medicine at Temple.

We counted 24 blocks flanking immediately or close to North Broad. Temple will tell you they have 17 schools and colleges, nine campuses, more than 400 degree programs, and approximately 38,000 students combine to create one of the nation's most diverse learning environments. It is the 31st-largest university and fourth-largest provider of professional education in the U.S.

Much of this operates within the Area of Influence of the William Penn Ley. Outside the Research Building the ley is three feet out on sidewalk..

The forecourt Temple Hospital is a couple of steps up from the street and is frequently graced by uniformed nurses and students seemingly from all parts of the world, standing, sitting and conversing, laughing, gesticulating and appearing so relaxed. Conwell and Penn would have loved it. Good things happen when Earth energy such as leys and geopirals abound and spread their influence.

Another great hospital on North Broad is Hahnemann University Hospital. This is another teaching hospital in the Center City region of Philadelphia. Established in 1885, it was named after Samuel Hahnemann, the founder of homeopathy. It is affiliated with Drexel University College of Medicine and serves as its Center City Hahnemann campus. It is also a Level One trauma center.

Hahnemann made Breaking News on August 3, 2000 when former President Gerald Ford was admitted to the hospital after suffering two minor strokes while attending the 2000 Republican National Convention. He made a quick recovery shortly afterwards.

One puzzling aspect of the North Broad Street area was the William Penn High School between Thompson and Master streets — yes, it occupied an entire block and was rated one of the best high schools in Pennsylvania. It closed in 2012.

Five buildings all connected by bridges formed a beautiful and majestic campus. At the peak of its prosperity there were so many students that street lines were put on the floors of major hallways to control student traffic. One building was divided in half to provide two full sized lunchrooms. The school included a childcare facility for students who were also parents. The top floor was a greenhouse. Up until 2006 it was operating at peak efficiency, then something happened. Within a handful of years enrolment declined to a mere 600 in 2011. The following year the school closed and when we came by in March 2016 bulldozers were turning it into history.

Before we leave North Broad, I have a personal memory. Back in 1978 when I lived in Vancouver, I studied metaphysics under British medium Patrick Young. One of the books he urged the students to acquire was Russell Conwell's *Acres of Diamonds*. It was one of those books that changed my life. While writing this section I downloaded the Kindle edition prepared for publication by Temple students and re-read it. A strange coincidence? Patrick used to say "There are no such things as coincidences: Just movements by Spirit for opportunities to learn."

In the opposite direction, South Broad Street holds a number of fascinating attractions for the artistically minded. For starters there is the Kimmel Center which is a world-class performing arts center. While we were there the new Broadway show *Beautiful: The Carol King Musical* was on for about two weeks and the next day from the Israel Film Festival the movie *A Tale of Love and Darkness* was being shown.

Also calling home on South Broad is the Meriam Theater, Academy of Music, the Arts Institute and the sprawling University of the Arts. Among its lengthy list of alumni is movie director Joe Dante *Gremlins I* and *II, The 'Burbs etc)*, actress Heather Donahue of the *Blair Witch Project*, actress, singer LaChanze who won a Tony Award for *Color Purple*, cartoonist and author Arnold Roth who created covers for The New Yorker and artwork in TV Guide, Sports Illustrated and Esquire. The list goes on.

One place that caught our dowsing and spiritual eye is the National Shrine of Saint Rita of Cascia which attracts thousands of visitors each year. A beautiful church with a declining congregation but a booming business in visits from pilgrims and sightseers.

St. Rita's can be found at 1166 South Broad. The visitor cannot miss the building because it is built in the style of a 14th century Renaissance church, complete with frescos, marble and stained glass, all in homage to St. Rita, a strange but heroic woman.

Born in 1381 in Roccaporena, a tiny village in the Umbrian Hills of Central Italy, Margherita was attracted to the local Augustinian nuns and wanted to join them but was rejected. So she became a wife, a mother and a widow. Her husband was murdered. In the last 15 years of her life, she became a nun and through her devotions brought about healing and a strange relationship with Jesus.

The story is that a thorn from the crown of Jesus pierced her forehead and the wound remained open and visible to the day of her death May 22, 1457 when the bells of the convent sounded, unaided by human hands. Known as St. Rita of Cascia, the habits she wore at the convent are encased in the Philadelphia shrine, which once served as a focal point for Italian immigrants. Today, bus loads of pilgrims and tourists from all over North America and places beyond visit the shrine.

Outside this sacred place on South Broad, the William Penn Ley travels down the middle of the street, where strange to say, cars are parked. Eventually the ley can be found on the east side of the street by the time it gets to the famous Philadelphia Naval Yard on the Delaware River.

The ley then crosses the river and passes through a place we have already visited, Soupy Island, a modern day children's plaground but a century ago a Sanitarium Playground for city kids seeking fresh air and good food in a bid to beat the scourge of tuberculosis.

# WILLIAM PENN AND CITY HALL

The William Penn Ley which stretches along North and South Broad Street in Philadelphia takes a break between the two and this is where the founder dictated that City Hall should stand: right on a triple-haired ley.

Located at 1 Penn Square, City Hall is the seat of government for the city of Philadelphia in the commonwealth of Pennsylvania. At 548 feet it was the tallest habitable building in the world as the 20th century dawned. Today, it is the state's 16th-tallest building. It is also big in other ways. It houses various branches of government, the Executive — the Mayor's Office, the Legislative — the City Council, and the Judicial Branch's Civil Courts — the Court of Common Pleas.

In 2007 the building was voted #21 on the American Institute of Architects' list of Americans' 150 favorite U.S. structures. Would you believe that over the years there have been calls for this great building to be torn down.

Designed by Scottish-born architect John McArthur, Jr., in the Second Empire style it was under construction from 1871 until 1901 at a cost of $24 million.

The folks at City Hall like to talk of records but here is one that is different. It could be the world's largest city hall that has a triple-haired ley line running through it.

Not only that, the statue of the fellow who figured everything out, stands on top of the building and the ley line. It is one of 250 sculptures created by Alexander Milne Calder that help create the uniqueness of the place Philadelphians calls City Hall.

Now something else. While Betty Lou and I were on location in Philadelphia we discovered another ley which runs across the William Penn Ley. Dowsers will find it on Market Street from one end to the other. It comes into City Hall and crosses the William Penn Ley on the south side of the Inner Courtyard at City Hall. We labeled it the Market Street Ley.

Besides two ley lines, there is also another energy generator built into City Hall. On the main roof there are eight very large pyramids stationed on corners and edges. They can only be seen from an aerial photo, a balloon, Google Earth or in part during a public visit to the City hall tower. When a pendulum is held over the Google Earth image or an aerial photo it immediately goes into a counter clockwise spin. Their compounded Area of Influence must be quite substantial.

When we tested it, the range was about six city blocks or half a mile. In other words, if a dowser armed with a pendulum focuses on City Hall anywhere with a half mile radius, the pendulum will swing counter-clockwise and refuse to swing clockwise.

In other words there is a predominance of Yin energies in downtown Philadelphia which is why many people live, work, invent and play in a laid back feminine energy.

At any one time a pedestrian can see two of the pyramids, so we wonder whose idea it was to add pyramid energy — Cosmic Principle energy — to City Hall. Did William Penn leave such instruction or was it the idea of the architect, John McArthur Jr.?

The William Penn Ley which extends across the Delaware into New Jersey, also heads north. After travelling along Broad Street which terminates at Cheltenham Aveue, they ley goes across Pennsylvania passing through the Nativity of Our Lord Church and School at Warminster and crossing the Delaware into New Jersey at the small community of Frenchtown.

FOR DOWSERS: William Penn Ley — 48 miles approx.
Coordinates are:
Soupy Island Playground, NJ. 39°52′35.74″ N 75°10′35.95″ W
Philadelphia Navy Yard (S Broad & Langley) 39°53′46.06″ N 75°10′33.01″ W
National Shrine of St. Rita 39°56′11.14″ N 75°10′01.27″ W
Philadelphia City Hall 39°57′09.78″ N 75°09′48.66″ W
Temple School of Medicine 40°00′24.48″ N 75°09′06.62″ W
North Broad & Cheltenham: 40°03′47.21″ N 75°08′22.01″ W
Warminster Cath.School: 40°12′20.96″ N 75°05′49.35″ W
Frenchtown (Bridge & Harrision) NJ: 40°31′35.32″ N 75°03′41.82″ W

# A PYRAMID OVER THE MARKET

As a dowser writing an informal leyline impact study I would like to have included some of the great places and organizations that call Market Street their home.

For instance there is the President's House, Philadelphia. This mansion at 6th & Market served as the presidential mansion for George Washington and John Adams. Philadelphia served as the temporary capital of the United States, 1790–1800, while the Federal City was under construction in the District of Columbia.

Also on Market Street is the Philadelphia Stock Exchange (PHLX), now known as NASDAQ OMX PHLX. It is the oldest stock exchange in the United States, founded in 1790. It moved into the ley zone at 19th and Market as late as 1981.

Drexel University butts into Market Street across from the Earle-Mack School of Law. The Biddle Law Library is just along the street plus at least a dozen churches, a handful of libraries, investment service offices and under all this, deep underground, runs the subway trains on SEPTA's Market — Frankford Line.

It all happens in spite of the gentle all-pervading Earth energy of the Market Street Ley which runs along the middle of Market. If you wish to dowse it, walk over to City Hall and Penn Square which stands in an island between Market and Broad Street.

And talking of City Hall the Market Street Ley passes right outside the office responsible for gifts and registering people for tours, such as taking the elevators — there are two — up to the observation floor right underneath the statue of William Penn. It is a mite claustrophobic and a little hairy if one is averse to heights, but otherwise the experience is magnificent. Philadelphia and Pennsylvania all on a carpet before you. Perhaps your elation is enhanced by the fact that both you and William Penn are standing on the the Broad Street ley. Enjoy!

After being on this journey of Chasing the Cosmic Principle, one is always on the alert for pyramids. They can sneak into one's life like a small ornament, a crystal, a layout like we saw on a sidewalk at Princeton

University, or the ones we saw on the tops of the obelisks, and the flock of eight positioned on the rooftop of Philadelphia City Hall, which as you stand on the Observation Deck is below you.

If you gaze west over Market Street you will see one. We first realized its existence while watching the Channel Seven, CBS news. A large pyramid in Philadelphia! It is one of the background shots for the meteorologists. It can also be seen on Google Earth from Space.

If you are a pedestrian outside 1735 Market Street the pyramid is out of sight. The BNY Mellon Center completed in 1990 soars 54 stories or almost 800 feet. It stands on the former site of the Philadelphia Greyhound Bus Terminal and is now an elegant office complex home to a bunch of leading edge financial companies.

The architects were the award-wining international team of Kohn, Pedersen Fox Associates who designed the controversial and unique Midfield Terminal Complex at Abu Dhabi International Airport in the Middle East which puts most US airports back in the cardboard box age.

Back to the Mellon Center. A ley runs along Market Street and there is a full blown pyramid on the roof, the 52$^{nd}$ floor of the building. What a great combination! And lo and behold, according to Wikipedia there is a private business group, the Pyramid Club strategically placed 52 floors high at the "top of the town," above Center City in Philadelphia. The Club specializes in outstanding cuisine, personalized service, superb meeting and dining facilities, and state-of-the-art technology and if the managers do not know it, waves of energy from the Cosmic Principle.

This is not a "show and tell" pyramid, the Area of Influence covers a radius of about eight city blocks. If one walks west with a pendulum and focuses on the pyramid it will influence the pendulum to swing counter-clockwise for quite a distance.

But wait says the alert dowser. Why west? If you walk east your pendulum is going to be under the influence of the eight City Hall pyramids which are also power houses of Cosmic energy. The strategy is to focus on the actual pyramid that you are measuring. Mellon Pyramid — focus on that. City Hall Pyramids — focus on those. It is a good place for a dowser to learn focusing. The practicing dowser soon finds the area is a power house for learning Earth energies, thanks to William Penn and King Charles II.

## FOR DOWSERS: MARKET STREET LEY

E stimated distance10 miles. If Market Street Ley is first picked up in the busy SEPTA Rail Yard at Millbourne. It travels east through a residential area before it picks up for a straight run on Market Street. Coordinates:
Septa Rail Yard, Millbourne: 39°57′47.48″ N 75°15′33.81″ W
Millbourne: Market St. 39°57′47.21″ N 75°14′57.63″ W
Schuylkill River Bridge: 39°57′16.54″ N 75°10′49.54″ W
Mellon Pyramid 39°57′11.63″ N 75°10′10.88″ W
City Hall Courtyard: 39°57′08.28″ N 75°09′48.58″ W
Market / 2nd St intersection by Delaware: 39°56′59.70″ N 75°08′37.50″ W
Camden City Hall, NJ: 39°56′41.79″ N 75°07′13.24″ W
The Market Street Ley goes through Penn's Landing, crosses the Delaware and (by coincidence?) passes directly through Camden City Hall, New Jersey.

## THINGS TO DO FOR ENQUIRING DOWSERS

G ettysburg PA — Survey leyline at Baltimore Pike/Colgrove Ave. intersection near National Military Park. Coordinates: 39°48′34.39″ N 77°13′08.37″ W

LEYS WITH A HISTORY: Find and plot leys and geospirals in your area. If you need practice acquire Google Earth and find one of the leys described in this book using the coordinates, if necessary. Get the "feel" with your pendulum. Then check your own area or favorite region. When you find something digitally, record the coordinates and travel to the exact spot and physically confirm. Keep records. Then, if you wish, investigate the history of the ley and any associated geospirals and people and events affected by them. This is called personalizing Earth energies and it may well surprise you. This offers a great learning experience for the investigating dowser and, in addition, the folks who read about dowsing Earth energies and the Cosmic Principle at home.

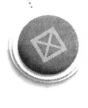

# THE FINALE

## PROVE IT TO YOURSELF

Chasing the Cosmic Principle is one of those strange, sometimes frustrating occupations but if one keeps a head above traditional logic, the pursuit often provokes new findings, new questions that frequently pose more tantalizing and even more frustrating questions. But it has often been said it is the experience gained on the journey that counts.

Even after trekking through home and foreign energy paths Betty Lou and I still have no good answer why certain things generate a counter clockwise spin of the pendulum. Not just a nice, comfortable spin but a vigorous ever building force.

We can never tire of asking why?

Even while I write this section there is word that a member of the British Society of Dowsers has noted that if a hiker walks counter-clockwise round a pyramid it is infinitely much easier than walking clockwise. So, I laid an eight inch drawing of the Cosmic Principle on the office floor and lo and behold there is some truth in this. Prove it to yourself.

Four good words — prove it to yourself. That is the message running through this notebook — do these things yourself. The energies are abundant and free if you have the incentive to test them.

Draw a Cosmic Principle four, five or eight inches, it matters not. Place it in your bedroom and see if it changes your sleeping habits. Positively? Make a note or keep a diary of any feelings, mental and physical and perhaps any dreams. Negatively? In your diary write what occurred in dreams, your feelings and if it is not for you, destroy the drawing, do not keep it around on a shelf, etc. It will keep working until destroyed. It is the same as decreeing a negative energy line for a workshop. Clean it up afterwards because it will keep working. In any case, please drop me a brief description of your experiences. Thinking further afield is this why so many pyramids were decapitated, not just for possible gold, but because someone knew of their powers?

If you possess an enquiring mind consider becoming an investigative dowser. People tell me they are a rare breed. With your pendulum test anything and everything and the moment your pendulum refuses to go clockwise and pulls to go counter-clockwise, you have something different to investigate.

As we mentioned earlier there is a strange phenomenon occuring with the Cosmic Principle. It started with pyramids of great size like the Great Pyramid at Giza and when a map or a diagram of a pyramid is made, the Cosmic Principle continues even with a miniature one or two inch pyramid.

What seems peculiar is that the Cosmic Principle, the square with a diagonal cross, like the pyramid has a distinct Area of Influence measuring more than ten or twenty times its own size and it radiates Yin energy, a peaceful, healthy, invigorating, inspirational energy.

But the counter-clockwise pendulum extends to other things. The famous sacred Aztec Sun Calendar in Mexico City has nothing that resembles the plan of a pyramid, yet its power insists a pendulum swing counter-clockwise. Why? Now, even more important, does this phenomenon of the counter-clockwise extend to other seemingly every day objects? Dowsers traditionally ask questions and receive responses. Now, if one holds a pendulum and stands over a pyramid or simply a plan of a pyramid without asking a question, there is a distinct reaction. The pendulum commences a counter-clockwise swing that just gets faster and faster.

Even more weird, if one walks away from the pyramid the pendulum continues to swing counter-clockwise until its Area of Influence ceases.

There seems to be a deeper meaning because this phenomenon is now found in other every day items.

Bernard suggested we test the pendulum over the printed "Elements Listed by Atomic Number." In eight out of 118 the pendulum insisted turning counter-clockwise and they are listed in these pages. There's a strong suggestion that most of the eight are connected to or are radioactive. Is it the word or is it the subject itself that causes this? There's work here for an enquiring dowser or an academic to discover the reasons.

Our experiments took us along a varied and totally unplanned course. We know that other things prompt a counter-clockwise spin: the so-called Cosmic Number "9" even written as "nine" triggers a counter-spin. When printed or written as an 18, 27, etc., which all reduce to nine, they have no effect.

Out of all the keys on a piano the C note commands a counter-spin. A C note on a flute does the same thing. Why?

Bernard popped up and said "Try an S." We found it is the only letter of the 26 letter alphabet that commands a counter-clockwise spin of the pendulum.

At this point we commenced tossing words at random under the pendulum like God, Allah, Taos, Cuneiform, Babylon, newspaper, television, Holy Bible, Buddha, Pharaoh, and more but the pendulum just swings clockwise. Boring stuff until we hit these words: Sacred, Letter, Arsenal and Love. All counter-clockwise! At this point, nothing made any logical sense.

Then we struck an anomaly. The word Spirit prompts a clockwise pendulum, but change the word into Spiritual and it goes counter-clockwise. Why?

Colors, what about colors? I put the question to Bernard.

"Yellow," he said easily. "Any way and in any language it fits the Cosmic Principle."

Among metaphysicians and some designers and artists yellow represents wisdom and in many cultures it represents sunshine, happiness and warmth. Betty Lou was wearing a yellow blouse that day. Counter-clockwise.

Bernard mentioned language. The English word Yellow is Amarillo in Spanish-speaking countries, Jaune in France, Gelb in Germany, and Kitrinos in Greece. What about Latin? Crocus. Yellow in any language prompts a counter-clockwise spin of the pendulum.

After some thought we decided it was not the word that prompts the counter-spin but the connection to the object itself. It was the Latin word Crocus that suggested the word "Sun" should be tested, after all, the sun is yellow.

Use a pendulum on the word Sun and watch what happens: A definite counter-spin. The next words examined: Star and Galaxy both produced clockwise spins but the Moon, Lunar and Solar-system returned a counter-spin.

If the color Yellow commands a counter-spin in different languages what do the languages themselves command in pendulum responses? There are 104 languages listed on Google Translate so we tested the entire list and the pendulum swung clockwise on all except three. They are English, Welsh and Tamil.

English stemmed from the original Indo-European but as no writings exist from that time, the very earliest examples of writing, Cuneiform, occurred in Sumeria about 6,000 years ago. Welsh or Cymraeg is the oldest language in Britain dating back well over 4,000 years, perhaps more. Tamil in South Asia is a language and culture that originated with the the Proto Dravidian language considered to have existed over 2,500 years ago.There is a movement to make it the language of the United Nations.

Betty Lou and I are very interested in the Basque culture and language. My historical novel *For the Love of Rose* is set for a major part in the Basque Country of Spain. Basque like Welsh and Tamil are ancient languages, so when the pendulum scanned the Google Translate language list the pendulum did not respond at "Basque"

Basques speak a language called Euskara or Euskadi. It is a pre-Indo-European language with roots originating in pre-historic times. It has no connection to any other in the world so we tested it. A definite counter-clockwise spin making four languages — English, Welsh, Euskadi and Tamil — in the Cosmic Principle.

For the Enquiring Dowser the motto should be: "If it seems Cosmic test it." Bearing this in mind, Betty Lou obtained a hefty Random House Webster's College Dictionary and armed with a pendulum asked it to show me a Yes if there was a Cosmic Principle word on the page being shown. I had no intention of performing a full word scan but intended to simply scan the pages of all words starting with the letter A.

There was some logic in this. I already knew the word Arsenal draws a counter-clockwise response, would the pendulum pick it up? As I flipped the pages every three or four seconds the pendulum gave a sharp tug at page 77. Using my pointer I slid it through the words quite quickly not even attempting to see or recognize any words. Suddenly the pendulum gave a hesitant counter-clockwise spin signifying something there. I looked and the pointer was two words words away from Arsenal. When the pointer was adjusted on Arsenal the pendulum went into a hard counter-spin.

All in all 99 pages with words starting with the letter A were scanned and only six words triggered a counter-spin. They were: Abacus, Agave, Antineutrino, Antipodes, Arsenal and Azimuth. We wondered, what would happen if we deleted the prefix Anti and left Neutrino? Both words bring about counter-spins. Anti responds clockwise.

And what is a Neutrino? The good guys at the University of California in Irvine — UCI.EDU — write: "Neutrinos are one of the fundamental particles which make up the universe. They are also one of the least understood. Neutrinos are similar to the more familiar electron, with one crucial difference: neutrinos do not carry electric charge."

Are the pyramids, the pendulums, the leys, the geospirals and the plan Spirit calls the Cosmic Principle trying to tell us something? There are some definite signposts. A dowser cabin-bound by ten feet of winter snow in the Adirondacks or the Rockies might scan the full dictionary and find a jumble of meaningless words or more importantly a critical message for the future of the Human Race.

So for any dedicated dowsers and would be questers who wish to take up thy rods, staffs and pendulums, keep on asking questions and maybe Chasing the Cosmic Principle will end in a blast of glorious enlightenment.

Blessings from the Old Track.

Robert Egby and Betty Lou Kishler

## INTERNET:

Nissan Pyramid 1978 Project in Egypt / youtube.com/watch?v=OHOgtQa7LVw

Great Pyramid of Giza Research Association / gizapyramid.com/

Cahokia Mounds Historic Site, Illinois / CahokiaMounds.org

Pierre Charles L'Enfant / arlingtoncemetery.net/l-enfant.htm

Waldorf School Princeton / princetonwaldorf.org/

Princeton Cemetery / wikipedia.org/wiki/Princeton_Cemetery

Colliers Mills WMA / nynjtc.org/park/colliers-mills-wildlife-management-area

Education Testing Services, Princeton NJ / ets.org

Chapin School, Princeton, NJ / chapinschool.org/history

Temple University, PA South Broad / temple.edu/

The National Shrine of St. Rita, South Broad / saintritashrine.org/

University of the Arts, Philadelphia / uarts.edu/

History Pine Ridge Cemetery, Saranac Lake, NY / https://localwiki.org/hsl/Pine_Ridge_Cemetery

The cured & uncured at Saranac Lake NY / localwiki.org/hsl/Famous_Visitors

The Pyramid at BYN Mellon Center, Philadelphia / en.wikipedia.org/wiki/BNY_Mellon_Center_(Philadelphia)

Baldy Town Boy Scouts / ghosttowns.com/states/nm/baldy.html

Inside the Great Pyramid / stevenhalpern.com/prod/meditation-music/initiation.html

Jefferson Lab / education.jlab.org/itselemental/index_num.html

Babylonian Clay Tablet YBC 7289 / en.wikipedia.org/wiki/Yale_Babylonian_Collection#/media/File:Ybc7289-bw.jpg

Pyramid Club, Philadelphia / clubcorp.com/Clubs/Pyramid-Club/

US History: Market Street / ushistory.org/philadelphia/street_market.htm

British Dowsers / britishdowsers.org/shop/

Maria Wheatley / theaveburyexperience.co.uk/index.html

American Society of Dowsers / dowsers.org/bookstore/

Canadian Society of Dowsers / canadiandowsers.org/

Canadian Society of Questers / questers.ca/

Pierre-François Réal / shannonselin.com/2014/12/pierre-francois-real/

Chittenango, NY All Things Oz Museum / oz-stravaganza.com/

Governors Island, NY / governorsislandalliance.org/history/

Governors Island, NY / nps.gov/gois/planyourvisit/directions.htm.

Soupy Island, NJ / jerseyfamilyfun.com/soupy-island-hidden-treasure-gloucester-county/

UCI.EDU — Neutrino / ps.uci.edu/~superk/neutrino.html

Philadelphia City Hall / phlvisitorcenter.com/attraction/city-hall-visitor-center/

Spiritualists at Lily Dale NY, / lilydaleassembly.com/

Earthship Biotecture, Taos, NM / earthship.com/

Sacred City of Caral, Peru / whc.unesco.org/en/list/1269

History of English Language / thehistoryofenglish.com/history_before.html

Babylonian Tablet YBC 7289 / math.ubc.ca/~cass/euclid/ybc/ybc.html

## BOOKS:

UFO EXPERIENCES IN CANADA by Vicki Cameron. General Store Publishing House. (highly recommended)

Einstein: The Life of a Genius, Walter Isaacson / Carlton Books

Acres of Diamonds by Russell Conwell / Tremendous Life Books

Earth Radiation by Käthe Bachler / John Living Publishing

The Ley Hunter's Companion by Paul Devereux & Ian Thomson / Thames & Hudson

The Essential Dowsing Guide by Dennis Wheatley. Celestial Songs Press

Early British Trackways by Alfred Watkins / Biblio Bazaar

The Pattern of the Past by Guy Underwood / Abelard-Schuman Ltd.

Earthship Earth: A Coming of Wizards by Michael E. Reynolds / Solar Survival Press

Emigrés in the Wilderness by T. Wood Clarke / Lewis & Clark

The Making of Urban America by John W. Reps / Princeton Univ. Press

Holy Dirt, Sacred Earth: A Dowser's Journey in New Mexico by Robert Egby / Three Mile Point Publishing

Tomb of Osiris: Encyclopedia of Ancient Egypt by Dr. Selim Hassan. 1944/Page 193

Notable Black American Women by Shirelle Phelps / Gale

The Philosophy of Freedom by Rudolph Steiner / Steiner

## NEWSPAPERS

NASA Evidence of Mysterious Ancient Earthworks. NY Times. Internat. Ed. 10/30/2015

## Non-fiction

CRACKING THE GLASS DARKLY: The Ancient Path to Lasting Happiness

THE QUEST OF THE RADICAL SPIRITUALIST: The Journey Begins

INSIGHTS: The Healing Paths of the Radical Spiritualist

HOLY DIRT, SACRED EARTH: A Dowser's Journey in New Mexico

CHASING THE COSMIC PRINCIPLE: Dowsing from Pyramids to Back Yard America

## Historical fiction

PENTADAKTYLOS: Love, Promises & Patriotism in the Last Days of Colonial Cyprus.

THE GUARDIANS OF STAVKA: The Deadly Hunt for the Romanov Gold

CATACLYSM '79: The Day the River Stopped

UNPLUGGED: The Return of the Fathers (historical sci-fi)

FOR THE LOVE OF ROSE: A Journey in Three Worlds

POR EL AMOR DE ROSE: Un Viaje en tres mundos (Spanish)

## Autobiography

KINGS, KILLERS & KINKS IN THE COSMOS: Treading Softly With Angels Among Minefields

CPSIA information can be obtained
at www.ICGtesting.com
Printed in the USA
FFOW02n0715141116
29309FF